Evolving Treatment Paradigms for Renal Cancer

Guest Editors

WILLIAM HUANG, MD
SAMIR S. TANEJA, MD

UROLOGIC CLINICS OF NORTH AMERICA

www.urologic.theclinics.com

Consulting Editor
SAMIR S. TANEJA, MD

May 2012 • Volume 39 • Number 2

SAUNDERS an imprint of ELSEVIER, Inc.

W.B. SAUNDERS COMPANY
A Division of Elsevier Inc.

1600 John F. Kennedy Blvd. • Suite 1800 • Philadelphia, PA 19103-2899

http://www.theclinics.com

UROLOGIC CLINICS OF NORTH AMERICA Volume 39, Number 2
May 2012 ISSN 0094-0143, ISBN-13: 978-1-4557-3949-3

Editor: Stephanie Donley

Urologic Clinics of North America (ISSN 0094-0143) is published quarterly by Elsevier Inc., 360 Park Avenue South, New York, NY 10010-1710. Months of issue are February, May, August, and November. Business and Editorial Offices: 1600 John F. Kennedy Blvd., Suite 1800, Philadelphia, PA 19103-2899. Periodicals postage paid at New York, NY and additional mailing offices. Subscription prices are $339.00 per year (US individuals), $561.00 per year (US institutions), $396.00 per year (Canadian individuals), $687.00 per year (Canadian institutions), $492.00 per year (foreign individuals), and $687.00 per year (foreign institutions). Foreign air speed delivery is included in all *Clinics* subscription prices. All prices are subject to change without notice. **POSTMASTER:** Send address changes to *Urologic Clinics of North America*, Elsevier Health Sciences Division, Subscription Customer Service, 3251 Riverport Lane, Maryland Heights, MO 63043. Customer Service: 1-800-654-2452 (US). From outside the United States, call 1-314-447-8871. Fax: 1-314-447-8029. E-mail: JournalsCustomerServiceusa@elsevier.com (for print support) and JournalsOnlineSupport-usa@elsevier.com (for online support).

Reprints. For copies of 100 or more, of articles in this publication, please contact the Commercial Reprints Department, Elsevier Inc., 360 Park Avenue South, New York, New York 10010-1710. Tel.: 212-633-3813; Fax: 212-462-1935; E-mail: reprints@elsevier.com.

Urologic Clinics of North America is covered in MEDLINE/PubMed (*Index Medicus*), *Excerpta Medica, Current Contents/Clinical Medicine, Science Citation Index,* and *ISI/BIOMED.*

Printed and bound by CPI Group (UK) Ltd, Croydon, CR0 4YY

Transferred to Digital Print 2012

Contributors

CONSULTING EDITOR

SAMIR S. TANEJA, MD
The James M. and Janet Riha Neissa Professor
of Urologic Oncology; Professor of Urology and
Radiology; Director, Division of Urologic
Oncology, Department of Urology, New York
University Langone Medical Center, New York
University Cancer Institute; Program Leader,
Genitourinary Oncology Program, New York
University Cancer Institute, New York,
New York

GUEST EDITORS

WILLIAM HUANG, MD
Assistant Professor, Department of Urology,
New York University Langone Medical Center,
New York University Cancer Institute,
New York, New York

SAMIR S. TANEJA, MD
The James M. and Janet Riha Neissa Professor
of Urologic Oncology; Professor of Urology and
Radiology; Director, Division of Urologic
Oncology, Department of Urology, New York
University Langone Medical Center, New York
University Cancer Institute; Program Leader,
Genitourinary Oncology Program, New York
University Cancer Institute, New York,
New York

AUTHORS

GENNADY BRATSLAVSKY, MD
Urologic Oncology Branch, National Cancer
Institute, National Institutes of Health,
Bethesda, Maryland; Professor and Chair,
Department of Urology, SUNY Upstate Medical
University, Syracuse, New York

JEFFREY A. CADEDDU, MD
Professor of Urology and Radiology,
Department of Urology, University of Texas
Southwestern Medical Center, Dallas, Texas

HERSH CHANDARANA, MD
Department of Radiology, New York
University Langone Medical Center,
New York, New York

FANG-MING DENG, MD, PhD
Department of Pathology, New York University
School of Medicine, New York, New York

CHRISTOPHER P. EVANS, MD
Professor and Chairman, Department of
Urology, University of California, Davis
Medical Center, Sacramento, California

STEPHEN FADDEGON, MD
Assistant Clinical Instructor, Department of
Urology, University of Texas Southwestern
Medical Center, Dallas, Texas

BRIAN HU, MD
Department of Urology, University of California,
Davis Medical Center, Sacramento, California

Contributors

WILLIAM HUANG, MD
Assistant Professor, Department of Urology,
New York University Langone Medical Center,
New York University Cancer Institute,
New York, New York

STELLA K. KANG, MD
Department of Radiology, New York University
Langone Medical Center, New York, New York

PATRICK A. KENNEY, MD
Fellow, Urologic Oncology, Department
of Urology, MD Anderson Cancer Center,
Houston, Texas

EMIL KHETERPAL, MD
Bruce Sherman Fellowship in Urologic
Oncology, Division of Urologic Oncology,
New York University Langone Medical Center,
New York, New York

SIMON P. KIM, MD, MPH
Department of Urology, Mayo Clinic,
Rochester, Minnesota

BRIAN R. LANE, MD, PhD
Spectrum Health Hospital System; Clinical
Associate Professor, Department of Surgery,
Michigan State University College of Human
Medicine; Adjunct Clinical Associate
Professor, Labarotories of Computational
Biology and Genetic Epidemiology, Van Andel
Research Institute, Grand Rapids, Michigan

PRIMO N. LARA JR, MD
Professor, Division of Hematology and
Oncology, Department of Internal Medicine,
School of Medicine, University of California,
Davis, Sacramento, California

JONATHAN MELAMED, MD
Department of Pathology, New York University
School of Medicine, New York, New York

BRIAN SHUCH, MD
Urologic Oncology Branch, National Cancer
Institute, National Institutes of Health,
Bethesda, Maryland

ERIC A. SINGER, MD, MA
Urologic Oncology Branch, National Cancer
Institute, National Institutes of Health,
Bethesda, Maryland

GANESH SIVARAJAN, MD
Department of Urology, New York University
Langone Medical Center, New York, New York

SAMIR S. TANEJA, MD
The James M. and Janet Riha Neissa Professor
of Urologic Oncology; Professor of Urology and
Radiology; Director, Division of Urologic
Oncology, Department of Urology, New York
University Langone Medical Center, New York
University Cancer Institute; Program Leader,
Genitourinary Oncology Program, New York
University Cancer Institute, New York,
New York

R. HOUSTON THOMPSON, MD
Department of Urology, Mayo Clinic,
Rochester, Minnesota

CHRISTOPHER M. WHELAN, MD
Spectrum Health Hospital System; Clinical
Assistant Professor, Department of Surgery,
Michigan State University College of Human
Medicine, Grand Rapids, Michigan

CHRISTOPHER G. WOOD, MD, FACS
Professor and Deputy Chairman, Department
of Urology, MD Anderson Cancer Center,
Houston, Texas

Contents

Each histologic type of renal cell carcinoma (RCC) has different pathologic and clinical parameters; however, the independent role of histologic type in outcome prediction remains contested. Most studies show relevance for outcome of each histologic type when correlated with survival by univariate analysis, whereas few studies show differences in outcome once other key prognostic factors, such as stage and grade, are considered. These studies highlight the challenges to prove outcome relevance. Despite the contested independent value of type for outcome prediction, separation of RCC into types is well accepted and can be substantiated on clinical, pathologic, molecular, and general outcome differences.

Although the management of sporadic renal tumors is challenging enough, dealing with those with bilateral, multifocal, and hereditary kidney cancer adds an additional level of complexity. A clinician managing this patient population must understand the hereditary syndromes and the genetic testing available. Treating physicians must be familiar with enucleative surgery, complex or multiple tumor partial nephrectomy, complex renal reconstruction, re-operative renal surgery, and active surveillance strategies. With proper management, most patients affected with bilateral, multifocal, or hereditary RCC can have a long life expectancy while maintaining adequate renal function.

Over the last two decades, there has been a rising incidence of renal tumors, particularly, small renal masses (<4 cm) resulting in a downward size and stage migration. This has brought about a paradigm shift in the management of newly diagnosed renal masses, such that nephron-sparing surgery, minimally invasive techniques, and active surveillance are frequently considered preferable to the historical gold standard of open radical nephrectomy. Population-based cohort studies indicate, however, that the widespread adoption of these techniques has been relatively slow and incomplete leading to significant disparities in the delivery of care throughout the country. Further investigation is required to determine the barriers to diffusion of new techniques and technology as well as to ensure equal access to quality care in the United States.

Localized kidney cancer is ideally managed with surgical extirpation. Historically renal cell carcinoma has been treated with radical nephrectomy, but partial nephrectomy has become increasingly used because of a growing body of evidence demonstrating equivalent oncologic control and a potential benefit in overall survival. In this article, the authors demonstrate that partial nephrectomy carries excellent oncologic efficacy. They additionally review the growing indications for partial nephrectomy and factors influencing candidate selection. The authors also compare the relative outcomes of open and minimally invasive techniques. Several factors influence outcome, and surgeon experience should dictate the choice of technique.

Proper integration of surgery and systemic therapy is essential for improving outcomes in renal cell carcinoma (RCC). There is no current role for adjuvant therapy after nephrectomy for clinically localized disease. The potential benefits of neoadjuvant therapy for locally advanced nonmetastatic disease are in need of further study. In metastatic disease, the proper integration of cytoreductive surgery and systemic therapy remains to be elucidated. Presurgical targeted therapy is feasible and may be beneficial. Pending the results of randomized controlled trials, upfront cytoreductive nephrectomy in appropriate patients will likely continue as the paradigm of choice in metastatic RCC.

Treatment of metastatic renal cell carcinoma (mRCC) has evolved dramatically within the past 10 years with the advent of therapy targeting the angiogenesis and mammalian target of rapamycin (mTOR) pathways. These therapies rapidly supplanted immunotherapy as a first-line systemic treatment option. Response rates, however, continue to vary, largely due to mRCC's clinical and molecular heterogeneity. This article reviews current understanding of mRCC biology and available treatments, discusses novel biomarkers that improve prognostication and may be able to predict response, and integrates available literature on surgical and systemic therapies into an individualized strategy.

Urologic Clinics of North America

THE CLINICS ARE NOW AVAILABLE ONLINE!

Access your subscription at:
www.theclinics.com

Foreword

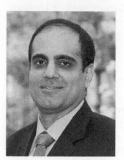

Samir S. Taneja, MD
Consulting Editor

Starting this year, I have agreed to take over as Consulting Editor for the *Urologic Clinics*. Many of you know that this position was previously held by Martin Resnick, someone who I considered to be a giant in our field since the time I was a student. As such, this is a great honor for me. The *Urologic Clinics of North America* has historically been a tremendous resource in American urology. During my training, this was the main source from which urologists gathered well-organized, condensed, up-to-date, information regarding focused topics in Urology.

Times are very different from when I was a resident, and now information is gathered, processed, and presented at a different rate. Most of our trainees, and practicing urologists, utilize web-based resources and electronic texts for learning and updating their knowledge base. As such, periodicals such as the *Urologic Clinics*, must strive to present information in a manner distinct from that which is widely available online. In keeping with this goal, the selected topics and authors must offer a unique perspective on the practice of Urology.

In taking on the role of consulting editor, I will make every effort to identify critical areas of rapid evolution in urologic practice and present them in a manner that is concise and useful. We will make an effort not just to provide information that is widely distributed, but to provide that information within specific context and with a thoughtful perspective, such that this information could be integrated into daily patient management. While this will be a challenge, I think it is feasible, and I am fully confident that the *Urologic Clinics* will continue to be a useful resource to us all. Throughout the process, I urge you all to communicate with me as often as you like to let me know how you feel about the content—and how you think we should evolve the content.

I am a firm believer in the transition of health care to multidisciplinary disease-based approaches. Urology will be a prime contributor to this model as we are truly organ-system experts. In this spirit, I plan to urge guest editors to develop content in a multidisciplinary manner such that our readers begin to think about the global impact of urologic diseases on patient health. In developing interdisciplinary strategies for dealing with disease, our current and future urologists should be leaders.

Urologists have always been technology "junkies," and this love has allowed our field to lead the charge in device development and implementation of technology in clinical care. As such, we will also devote an issue each year to advances in technology that have an immediate impact in our practice.

In this issue entitled *Evolving Treatment Paradigms for Renal Cancer*, I have served as co-guest editor along with my respected colleague, Dr William Huang. In constructing the issue, we have attempted to offer unique perspectives

Urol Clin N Am 39 (2012) xi–xii
doi:10.1016/j.ucl.2012.03.001

on a common topic. The articles have been constructed to reflect a multidisciplinary thought process regarding management of patients with renal cancer, inclusive of pathologic, genetic, radiologic, epidemiologic, medical, and, of course, surgical thought processes that should be enlisted in deciding on an individualized plan of care. We hope you will find this, and the fantastic forthcoming issues, to be of great use in the care of your patients.

Samir S. Taneja, MD
Division of Urologic Oncology
Department of Urology
NYU Langone Medical Center
NYU Cancer Institute
150 East 32nd Street
New York, NY 10016, USA

E-mail address:
samir.taneja@nyumc.org

Preface
Evolving Treatment Paradigms for Renal Cancer

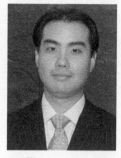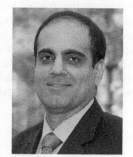

William Huang, MD   Samir S. Taneja, MD
Guest Editors

Over the past decade there have been steady advancements in the diagnosis, understanding, and management of renal cancers. While the mainstay of urologic therapy for both early- and late-stage disease remains surgery, new concepts in surgical management, novel therapeutic agents, and improved surgical technique have made treatment planning a more informed, multifactorial process. As such, despite the continued utilization of surgical therapy, the treatment paradigms utilized today have evolved considerably from those over the previous decade.

The story of renal cancer is progressively becoming similar to the story of another urologic malignancy—prostate cancer. Although we do not screen for kidney cancer, the liberal use of imaging has contributed to a steady increase in the incidence of renal cancer, with a subsequent downward size and stage migration. With an increased understanding of the natural history of the disease as well as the improvements in imaging and diagnostic techniques, there has been a realization that every newly diagnosed tumor does not necessarily require treatment. While long-term outcomes of renal surgery were not previously considered, the current demonstration of the significance of long-term renal functional outcomes has drawn another parallel with the considerations in prostate cancer surgery. The argument for conservative management of kidney cancers may be even more compelling than that of prostate cancer, given an increased understanding of the morbidity of

surgical treatment of renal cancers on kidney functional and other important nononcologic outcomes.

In this issue, it is our desire to demonstrate the multifactorial, multidisciplinary thought process involved in the contemporary management of the renal mass. Given the variable biological behavior of renal cancers, the paradigm of removing a mass simply because it is identified should no longer be part of the urologist's practice.

While evolution of the treatment paradigm for renal cancer has evolved in many ways, in this issue, we focus on a few particular themes. First, we attempt to create an evidence-based methodological approach to the small renal mass. In the article by Kang and colleagues, the authors discuss novel imaging approaches that may tell us something about the tumor before we biopsy or remove it. As imaging technology continues to provide more tumor-specific diagnostic information, treatment plans become individualized to the patient and tumor. The article by Deng and coworkers, on the significance of the histology of renal cancers, should allow an understanding of the variable biology of the disease. Finally, the article by Kim and colleagues provide a cohesive strategy for approaching the small renal mass at the time of diagnosis.

A second theme of the issue is that of surgical planning and the number of factors that currently go into the selection of the treatment approach. Once the decision for treatment is made, both host factors and tumor-related factors must be

Urol Clin N Am 39 (2012) xiii–xiv
doi:10.1016/j.ucl.2012.02.004

considered in developing an optimal individual approach to the tumor. In the article by Sivarajan and coworkers, current treatment trends in the utilization of nephron-sparing and minimally invasive procedures, as well as factors driving utilization, are reviewed. The article by Shuch and colleagues discusses the management of multifocal tumors, and the article by Lane and coworkers discusses the influence of individual treatment strategies on renal function and offers advice on how this information should be used in selecting the surgical approach. The articles by Kheterpal and colleagues and Faddegon and colleagues review the outcomes of various nephron-sparing approaches.

The final theme of this issue is to define a role for the urologist in the management of advanced renal cell carcinoma. The recent FDA approval of a number of biologic agents, efficacious in the treatment of metastatic disease, has rejuvenated the interest of medical oncologists in kidney cancer. It remains of critical importance that urologists maintain a firm grounding in their knowledge of available agents, factors influencing treatment, and the role of surgery within a multidisciplinary treatment strategy. In the article by Kenney and coworkers, the role of surgery in the era of tyrosine kinase inhibitors is discussed, and in the article by Hu and coworkers, a comprehensive individualized strategy for advanced disease is suggested. The introduction of new agents into the management of advanced disease has brought with it many questions regarding sequence of therapy, selection of agent, and the role of surgery. We are confident that these articles will be helpful in guiding the reader through these complex issues.

As guest editors of this issue, our goal was to provide the reader with a valuable resource which familiarizes the reader with the current thinking and decision-making thought processes that have evolved over time for the treatment of all stages of renal cancer. We are extremely grateful for the hard work and effort of the authors of this issue. As recognized leaders in this field, their time is appreciated and their insight is invaluable.

William Huang, MD
Department of Urology
NYU Langone Medical Center
NYU Cancer Institute
150 East 32nd Street
New York, NY 10016, USA

Samir S. Taneja, MD
Division of Urologic Oncology
Department of Urology
NYU Langone Medical Center
NYU Cancer Institute
150 East 32nd Street
New York, NY 10016, USA

E-mail addresses:
William.Huang@nyumc.org (W. Huang)
Samir.Taneja@nyumc.org (S.S. Taneja)

Histologic Variants of Renal Cell Carcinoma: Does Tumor Type Influence Outcome?

Fang-Ming Deng, MD, PhD, Jonathan Melamed, MD*

KEYWORDS

- Renal cell carcinoma • Histologic type • Outcome
- Chromophobe renal cell carcinoma
- Papillary renal cell carcinoma
- Unclassified renal cell carcinoma
- Collecting duct carcinoma

Each type of renal cell carcinoma (RCC) shows differences in pathologic and clinical parameters, including prognostic relevance; however, the outcome prediction for each type remains controversial. In general, chromophobe and papillary RCC have been associated with more favorable outcomes than clear cell RCC, whereas those of collecting duct and unclassified types have been less favorable. Large series examining outcomes have shown prognostic significance of histologic types by univariate analysis; however, only a few series retain prognostic significance on multivariate analysis. The studies in which histologic type retains prognostic significance are single-institution studies with standardized assignment of histologic type. In contrast, multi-institutional studies or pooled data sets do not show independent prognostic significance of histologic type nor do smaller series from single institutions in which statistical strength is underpowered. Data on outcomes are more recently determined through evaluation of histologic types separately against matched clear cell types or accrued through pooled data sets. This article summarizes the outcomes data for chromophobe, papillary, collecting duct, and unclassified RCC, and also reviews the impact of histologic type on patients with metastatic RCC. As greater knowledge on RCC is gained, newer entities are emerging that may shift distribution of cases. Despite the contested role of histologic type as an independent predictor of outcome, separation of RCC into types is now well accepted and substantiated in clinical, biologic, molecular, and sometimes also in outcome differences.

RENAL CELL CARCINOMA CLASSIFICATION AND OTHER PROGNOSTIC FACTORS

The current 2004 World Health Organization (WHO) classification of renal cell carcinoma (RCC)[1] follows on the earlier Heidelberg[2] and Rochester classifications,[3] which in turn represent expansions of the Mainz classification.[4] The current classification recognizes the heterogeneity of RCC and describes distinct types of RCC with unique morphologic and genetic characteristics. The major histologic variants of RCC are clear cell, papillary, chromophobe, and collecting duct, and account for 90% to 95% of RCCs (**Table 1**). The classification also includes the less commonly encountered types of renal medullary carcinoma, Xp11 translocation carcinoma, carcinoma associated with neuroblastoma, and mucinous, tubular, and spindle cell carcinomas. An important category included within the classification is the unclassified type, which is assigned when a tumor does not readily fit into any other group.

In determining the prognostic strength of this classification system, one should recognize that it is already in its eighth year since publication

Department of Pathology, New York University School of Medicine, 560 First Avenue, New York, NY 10016, USA
* Corresponding author.
E-mail address: melamj01@nyumc.org

Urol Clin N Am 39 (2012) 119–132
doi:10.1016/j.ucl.2012.02.001
0094-0143/12/$ – see front matter © 2012 Elsevier Inc. All rights reserved.

Table 1
WHO 2004 classification: RCC type versus proportion of cases and generalizations on outcome to date

RCC Subtype	Proportion (%)	Outcome vs Clear Cell RCC
Clear cell RCC	80	—
Papillary RCC	10	Favorable
Chromophobe RCC	5	Favorable
Collecting duct	1	Unfavorable
RCC, unclassified	4–6	Unfavorable
Multilocular clear cell RCC	Exact proportion undetermined	Low malignant potential
Renal medullary carcinoma	but rare tumors likely to	Highly aggressive
Xp11 translocation carcinoma	account for <2% of tumors	Undetermined
Carcinoma associated with neuroblastoma	overall	Similar to clear cell RCC
Mucinous tubular and spindle cell carcinoma		Favorable with exception

and likely to be updated in the near future to incorporate additional emerging entities within the classification of RCC (**Table 2**). The impact of newer types on the overall proportion of cases within each type is uncertain, although it may be low because of the rarity of these emerging entities.

In evaluating studies on outcome, one should realize that the overwhelming group, clear cell RCC, is likely to disproportionately outweigh all other groups in studies subject to statistical analysis. Furthermore, a comparison of other newly introduced and rarely encountered types within the classification is limited by insufficient accumulated data and the small number of cases in each type. Inferences on the behavior of these newer types are insufficient for conclusive determination as are based on case reports or small series data.

The prognostic utility of histologic type as an independent prognostic factor remains debated, with some convinced of its value and others not. The current *American Joint Committee on Cancer* (*AJCC*) *Staging Manual* (7th edition), used routinely to characterize tumors, recommends the use of the WHO 2004 classification, stating that "the more common histopathologic types have distinct molecular characteristics and are associated with prognostic or predictive significance as reflected by their integration in predictive algorithms for RCC."[5] This statement about the prognostic impact of histopathologic type reflects a view that may not be widely accepted. This article further evaluates this issue.

To understand the role of histopathologic subtype, one must be aware of its value in the context of other recognized prognostic factors in RCC. Prognostic factors may be subdivided into (1) anatomic (TNM stage, tumor size), (2) histopathologic (nuclear grade and histologic subtype), and (3) clinical (symptoms and performance status; laboratory results). Of these factors, pathologic stage and nuclear grade represent the major prognostic variables used routinely in localized RCC.

Table 2
Newer entities since WHO 2004 classification

RCC Subtype	Prevalence	Outcome Relevance
Tubulocystic carcinoma	Rare	Not fully determined
Thyroid-like (follicular) renal carcinoma	Rare	Not fully determined
Acquired cystic disease-associated RCC/carcinoma associated with end-stage renal disease	Rare	Not fully determined
Clear cell papillary RCC	Rare	Not fully determined
Oncocytic papillary RCC	Rare	Not fully determined
Leiomyomatous RCC	Rare	Not fully determined

Increasingly, other prognostic variables have been added to stage and grade to improve predictive strength.

The role of stage as defined in the TNM classification is widely accepted and has been well validated as a key prognostic parameter in RCC.[6] With higher stage, including lymph node invasion and metastasis to other organs, patients have a progressively worse prognosis and shorter survival. The TNM system which defines stage is progressively modified to incorporate new evidence and is most recently revised in the AJCC 7th edition, released in 2010.[5] The TNM classification denotes that risk of malignancy increases with size. Frank and colleagues[7] have validated this showing that for each 1-cm increase, the likelihood of malignancy and high grade features in renal tumors increases. More recently, size has been shown to correspond with higher grade, with a 0% incidence of high-grade features in tumors smaller than 1 cm, increasing to a 59% incidence in tumors larger than 7 cm.[8]

Nuclear grade as described in the Fuhrman system is the most commonly used grading scheme for RCC, and has been shown in multiple prior studies to correlate with tumor size, stage, and metastasis in clear cell type RCC. Its role in papillary and chromophobe RCC is not widely accepted and has been questioned. Recently, newer nuclear grading schemes for chromophobe and papillary RCC have been proposed and await validation.[9–11]

Other histologic features include coagulative tumor necrosis and sarcomatoid transformation, which have been proven to be independent predictors of adverse outcome in clear cell RCC.[12] Sarcomatoid transformation, once considered a distinct subtype, is now recognized as a high-grade dedifferentiation that may occur in any subtype of RCC. It is characterized by spindle cell morphology, often with marked nuclear pleomorphism, and occurs in a minority (<5%) of all RCC. It is associated with higher stage and worse prognosis, resulting in a 5-year disease-specific survival of 22% compared with 79% in tumors without sarcomatoid transformation.[13]

HISTOLOGIC TYPE OF RCC: MORPHOLOGIC, CLINICAL, AND MOLECULAR FEATURES OF EACH TYPE
Clear Cell RCC

Clear cell RCC is defined (WHO 2004) as a malignant renal neoplasm composed of cells with a clear or eosinophilic cytoplasm within a delicate vascular network.[14] The typical tumor is solid with a golden yellow appearance (**Fig. 1**), and microscopically shows neoplastic cells that may be clear or eosinophilic when higher grade. Approximately one-third of all patients have metastatic disease at initial presentation, and 20% to 40% experience local recurrence or distant metastasis after nephrectomy.[15,16] The molecular/genetic clear cell RCC pathogenesis is based on two key molecular pathways: the hypoxia-inducible pathway associated with mutation of the Von Hippel-Lindau (VHL) tumor suppressor gene, and the mammalian target of rapamycin (mTOR) signaling pathway.

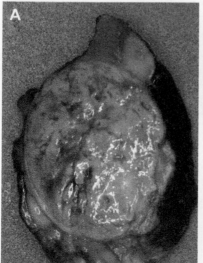 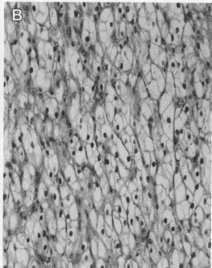

Fig. 1. Clear cell RCC. (*A*) Gross appearance as a well-circumscribed solid mass with golden yellow color. (*B*) Microscopic appearance shows tumor cells with clear cytoplasm and rich vascular network (hematoxylin-eosin stain, original magnification ×200).

Papillary RCC

Papillary RCC accounts for approximately 10% of all RCC and nearly 29% of RCC in African Americans. On macroscopic examination, these tumors are well circumscribed, often with a fibrous pseudocapsule,[17] and have a variegated appearance ranging from streaked dull yellow to uniformly dark brown (**Fig. 2**). Microscopically, the tumors show papillary or tubular architecture and occasionally may be solid. In the WHO classification, two types of papillary RCC are described: type 1, in which the neoplastic cells lining the cores are small with scant cytoplasm, and type 2, in which the cells are of higher nuclear grade with prominent nucleoli and have eosinophilic cytoplasm. The molecular pathway, different from that of clear cell type, also differs between types 1 and 2. In type 1, mutations of the MET oncogene (on chromosome 7) result in activation of the intracytoplasmic tyrosine kinase domains, which activate the hepatocyte growth factor pathway. The molecular pathway of type 2 is still to be fully elucidated but is suggested to be similar to that of the familial syndrome of hereditary leiomyomatosis and renal cell carcinoma, with a mutation in the fumarate hydratase gene (on chromosome 1). This results in upregulation of hypoxia-inducible factors (proangiogenic and growth factors).

Chromophobe RCC

Chromophobe RCC accounts for approximately 5% of surgically removed renal epithelial tumors, and typically has a pale tan appearance (**Fig. 3**). Thoenes and colleagues[18] first described this entity in 1985, showing a 4.6% incidence in a series of 697 RCC cases. Microscopically, it is characterized by a solid pattern of large polygonal cells with transparent reticulated cytoplasm, prominent cell membranes, wrinkled nuclei, and perinuclear halos. In the series to date, most tumors have been confined to the kidney; however, a small number (<5%) may present with metastasis or show sarcomatoid transformation. Insight on the molecular pathway driving these tumors is suggested from study of the Birt-Hogg-Dube syndrome, a hereditary form of this tumor in which there are frequently multifocal and bilateral tumors. The Birt-Hogg-Dube gene (on chromosome 17) produces a protein folliculin, which functions as a tumor suppressor and may activate the mTOR pathway.

Collecting Duct Carcinoma

Collecting duct carcinoma is a rare subtype of RCC, accounting for less than 2% of RCC (range, 0.4%–1.8%). Based on limited earlier evidence in the literature (case reports and small case series), these tumors are recognized to be highly aggressive, often presenting at advanced stage and resulting in a poor prognosis. They have been described as occurring in a wide patient age range, with a male predominance of approximately 2:1. These tumors are usually large when diagnosed and have a firm white to gray appearance, with irregular borders and areas of necrosis. The histologic features show an infiltrative tubular or

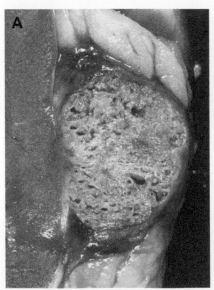
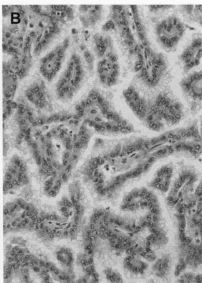

Fig. 2. Papillary RCC. (*A*) Gross appearance as a well circumscribed solid mass with variegated dull yellow color. (*B*) Microscopic appearance shows papillary architecture. The papillae are lined with a single layer of cells with scant cytoplasm and low-grade nucleus (type 1) (hematoxylin-eosin stain, original magnification ×200).

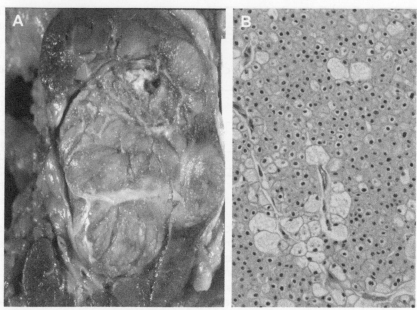

Fig. 3. Chromophobe RCC. (*A*) Gross appearance as a lobulated gray to brown solid mass. (*B*) Microscopic appearance shows tumor cells with sharp defined cell borders and perinuclear clearing (hematoxylin-eosin stain, original magnification ×200).

tubulopapillary pattern, associated with a desmoplastic stromal reaction, and frequent high nuclear grade (**Fig. 4**). The molecular pathway underlying CDC is poorly understood. Cytogenetic abnormailities include monosomy of chromosomes 1, 6, 14, 15 and 22 with allelic loss on chromosomal arms 1q, 6p, 8p, 13q, and 21q. A minimal deletion located at 1q32.1–32.2 was mapped in up to two thirds of CDC suggesting a tumor suppressor gene in this region.

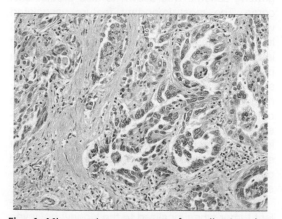

Fig. 4. Microscopic appearance of a collecting duct carcinoma showing tubulopapillary architecture with high grade tumor cells in a desmoplastic stroma (hematoxylin-eosin stain, original magnification ×200).

Unclassified RCC Category

The unclassified RCC category is a diagnostic category, not a specific type, and is used to assign RCCs that do not fit into the other RCC types based on histologic evaluation. It is recognized to be a heterogeneous group that therefore cannot be defined in a limited manner. Features that may cause a carcinoma to be placed in this category include a composite of other RCC subtypes, sarcomatoid morphology without recognizable epithelial elements, mucin production, mixtures of epithelial and stromal elements, and unrecognizable cell types. The assignment to this category varies from 0.7% to 5.7% in published series, reflecting varied criteria. Differences in outcome across series may be partly attributed to the definition used for unclassified RCC.

OUTCOMES DATA BASED ON SERIES OF INDIVIDUAL HISTOLOGIC TYPES OF NON–CLEAR CELL COMPARED WITH CLEAR CELL RCC

Papillary RCC: Outcome with Focus on Type 1 Versus Type 2

Outcome of papillary RCC has been recently evaluated in several large series (**Table 3**). These studies show that papillary RCC has a low risk of recurrence and cancer-related death after surgery (5-year survival, 86%–92%). Although prior studies showed

Table 3
Findings in several large cohorts of papillary RCC

Author	Cases	5-y Disease-Specific Survival (%)	Univariate Association of Type with Death	Multivariate Associations with Death
Zucchi et al,[46] 2011	577	86	Not assessed	N, M stage, Fuhrman nuclear grade
Klatte et al,[19] 2010	435	88.1	Type 1, 2 association	T, M stage, vascular invasion, necrosis, symptoms
Sukov et al,[47] 2012	395	91.8	Type 1, 2 association	T, N, M stage, grade

papillary carcinoma subtype to be of prognostic significance (type 2 having a worse prognosis than type 1) on both univariate and multivariate analysis in which stage is included, this has not been confirmed by several groups in subsequent studies. Several reasons have been proposed for these discrepant findings. These differences may relate to the difficulty in classification encountered when an overlap occurs between both subtypes (up to 35% tumors), the limit in statistical power in some studies because of small sample size and infrequency of death, and because earlier studies of papillary RCC used death from any cause rather than cancer-specific death to determine outcome relevance. In two of the three studies (see **Table 3**) evaluating type against outcome, papillary RCC type 1 versus 2 did not show a significant association with outcome on multivariate analysis. Instead, Fuhrman nuclear grade was associated with outcome. Other predictive factors on multivariate analysis were incidental detection, TNM stage, vascular invasion, and tumor necrosis extent. A nomogram for predicting outcome in papillary RCC was recently developed based on these other factors alone,[19] because subtyping into type 1 versus 2 did not merit inclusion. In a meta-analysis of eight studies of papillary RCC (totaling 309 papillary type 1 and 325 papillary type 2), Lee and colleagues[20] found type 2 to be associated with a lower survival rate on univariate analysis and, in studies in which multivariate data were available (totaling 438 cases), also found type 2 to be associated with lower survival on multivariate analysis.

Papillary RCC has an overall low risk of tumor recurrence and cancer death after nephrectomy; however, predictors of outcome relate to stage and nuclear grade. Although type of papillary RCC has been suggested as a prognostic factor, it is not validated in more recent larger series. Nevertheless, based on genetic differences, identification of types 1 and 2 papillary RCC should

continue to allow a better understanding of each subtype, even though its role for prognostic determination is currently debated.

Chromophobe RCC

In the past 4 years, several series have examined chromophobe type RCC in large number (**Table 4**), and have confirmed its favorable outcome. In the largest single-institution series to date, Przybycin and colleagues[21] show that these tumors are generally indolent, with only 4% developing recurrence or metastasis (>6-year median follow-up). Most of the tumors in this study were low stage (78%), with only a small proportion of chromophobe RCCs that subsequently recurred or metastasized. Histologic features associated with adverse outcome included tumor size, microscopic tumor necrosis, and sarcomatoid features. Nuclear grade did not show association with outcome. In another large series,[22] similarly histologic features, including tumor stage, were associated with adverse outcome; however, a modified nuclear grading scheme was shown to also predict outcome. The most important feature associated with adverse outcome in chromophobe RCC is sarcomatoid transformation which, although infrequent is disproportionately associated with metastasis or local recurrence. In another recent series from Korea with different sampling (larger number of high-stage and high-grade cases), the outcome was similar to clear cell RCC. In conclusion, localized chromophobe RCC remains an indolent tumor with excellent survival in most series; however, in some it may not show as good outcomes, related partly to case selection (inclusion of greater number of metastatic cases).

In conclusion, chromophobe RCC is an indolent tumor when localized to the kidney; however, when combined with metastatic cases, chromophobe RCC may not show any better outcome than clear cell RCC.

Table 4
Chromophobe RCC: outcome and prognostic factors

Author	Cases	5-y Disease-Specific Survival (%)	Metastasis (%)	Sarcomatoid Differentiation (%)	Association Analysis
Przybycin et al,[21] 2011	200	96.3	3.7 (after nephrectomy) + 2.5 (at presentation)	<2	Size >7 cm, tumor necrosis, sarcomatoid features, small vessel invasion
Amin et al,[22] 2008	145	NA	15 (after nephrectomy) + 3 (at presentation)	8	Sarcomatoid features, necrosis, T stage
Klatte et al,[48] 2008	124	78/91[a]	? (after nephrectomy) + 16 (at presentation)	15	Sarcomatoid features, TNM stage, Fuhrman grade, symptoms
Volpe et al,[49] 2011	291	93	8.6 (after nephrectomy) + 1.4 (at presentation)	1.8	Gender, T stage
Lee et al,[50] 2010	148	88.8	9.5	Not specified	—

[a] Nonmetastatic at presentation.

Collecting Duct Carcinoma

Most previous reports on collecting duct carcinoma have been limited to small numbers, which has precluded reliable statements on outcome. Recent pooled analyses of data have allowed study of large number of cases and provided a clearer picture of the clinical behavior of these tumors (**Table 5**). These studies show that it presents at a higher stage than clear cell RCC and is associated with worse disease-specific survival rates (70%–86% at 1 year and 45%–68% at 3 years). The largest series (from the United States)[23] found a twofold higher risk of death when compared with a matched clear cell RCC cohort, independent of grade and stage. These data showing a more adverse prognosis than for clear cell type are not corroborated in the European series. Possible explanations relate to misclassification of cases; the cases in the European series derived from an earlier period than those of the U.S. series, when diagnostic criteria may have differed.[24] The potential for misclassification is high, as shown in the Japanese series, in which centralized uropathology review showed misclassification in up to 33% of cases, potentially causing a dilution of adverse effect.

Unclassified RCC

In four of the largest series evaluating outcome, a total of 38 (Mayo Clinic), 85 (European), 31 (University of California, Los Angeles), and 23 (Henry Ford Hospital) cases were evaluated, in which the proportions assigned to the category of unclassified RCC were 1%, 1.3%, 2.8%, and 5.7% (**Table 6**). All series show that these tumors are usually high grade and high stage with a poor outcome. In the series by Amin and colleagues,[25] no difference in survival was seen on multivariate analysis, which may be attributed to small sample size lacking sufficient strength for true significance

to be tested. Zisman and colleagues[26] found an adverse impact on survival independent of stage and grade. Additionally, in a multi-institutional study, Karakiewicz and colleagues[27] compared 85 patients with unclassified RCCs versus 4322 with clear cell RCC, all of whom underwent nephrectomy. A matched analysis of patients with unclassified and clear cell RCC found a significant difference between survival rates (41% and 55%, respectively). The most recent series by Crispen and colleagues[28] similarly shows these tumors are likely to present with adverse prognostic features, such as advanced grade and stage, tumor necrosis, and sarcomatoid differentiation. When these cases were matched with clear cell RCC, however, no difference in outcome was seen. This single-institution series (Mayo Clinic) mostly consisted of cases of tumors with oncocytic features and high-grade malignant features (26 of 38). This assignment may differ from those in other series.

In conclusion, unclassified type is more likely than clear cell RCC to present with high stage and grade at diagnosis and has a higher proportion with sarcomatoid features and necrosis, and therefore is associated with a poor prognosis. When taking into account all adverse prognostic features, whether this category portends any worse prognosis remains unclear. It is important for pathologists to not lump low-grade tumors such as oncocytic tumors that are indeterminate between oncocytoma and chromophobe RCC into this category. More updated classifications will likely provide a better definition of this category to assure a more uniform group.

OUTCOME DATA IN LESS COMMON TYPES

The less-common types of translocation carcinoma, renal medullary carcinoma, neuroblastoma-associated RCC, mucinous tubular and spindle

---

Table 5
Collecting duct RCC: outcome and prognostic factors

Author	Cases	Disease-Specific Survival (%)	Metastasis[a] (Lymph node/ Distant) (%)	High Nuclear Grade/Poorly Differentiated (%)	Prognostic Association When Matched with Clear Cell RCC
Karakiewicz et al,[24] 2007	41	48 (5-y)	48.8/19.5	78	No difference
Tokuda et al,[51] 2006	81	34.3 (5-y)	44.2/32.1	97.5	Not available
Wright et al,[23] 2009	160	58 (3-y)	15[b]/28	70	Worse prognosis

[a] At presentation.
[b] In 77% lymph node status unavailable.

Table 6
Unclassified RCC: series evaluating outcome and prognostic factors

Author	Cases	Proportion	pT3 and pT4 (%)	M1 (%)	Sarcomatoid/ Tumor Necrosis	5-y Survival (Unclassified vs Clear Cell RCC)	Adverse Prognosis on Matched Multivariate Analysis
Zisman et al,[26] 2002	31 (1087)	2.8%	100%	94%	Not specified	Not provided (only 1 of 31 alive at 18.5 mo)	Yes
Amin et al,[25] 2002	23 (405)	5.7%	84.3%	69.6%	26%/not specified	24% vs 76%	No
Karakiewicz et al,[27] 2007	85 (6530)	1.3%	70.6%	54.1%	Not specified	36% vs 74.3%	Yes
Crispen et al,[28] 2010	38 (3085)	1%	(39.5%)	21%	24%/76%	43% vs 63% unmatched vs 47% matched	No

cell carcinoma have been newly introduced and lack sufficient data for analysis compared with clear cell RCC. Nevertheless, some trends in outcome may be used to subdivide these groups according to probable prognosis.

Multilocular clear cell RCC (MCRCC) is a tumor that is entirely cystic without a solid expansile component. As with classic clear cell RCC, the neoplastic cells show loss of 3p, suggesting that this type is a variant of clear cell RCC. It is separated into a different type, probably because of its marked difference in outcome. Unlike clear cell RCC, MCRCC has not been shown to ever metastasize, suggesting that this should be designated as a tumor of low malignant potential.[29]

Mucinous tubular and spindle cell carcinoma (MTSCC) is an uncommon type with female predominance (4:1). Genetic studies are few, with multiple genetic abnormalities detected through either comparative genomic hybridization or fluorescence in situ hybridization analyses, including losses of chromosomes 1, 4, 6, 8, 9, 13, 14, 15, and 22, and gains of chromosomes 7, 12q, 16q, 17, and 20q. The prognosis seems to be favorable for most MTSCCs. They are usually low grade, low stage, indolent, and cured with surgery, with low rate of recurrence and metastasis. Rare case reports exist of renal MTSCC with intraabdominal recurrences and regional lymph node metastases. More recently, case reports describe MTSCC with sarcomatoid change that resulted in distant metastases and rapidly fatal clinical courses. MTSCCs with classical morphology showing extensive metastasis have also been reported.

Neuroblastoma-associated RCC occur in young patients (median age, 13.5 years) and are morphologically heterogeneous, with some showing papillary architecture and others having clear cell features. The prognosis correlates with stage and grade similar to other types of RCC.

Translocation carcinoma is an uncommon subtype of RCC that harbors a translocation involving a member of the microphthalmia transcription factor gene family. These translocations most commonly involve the *TFE3* gene on locus Xp11.2, and less commonly involve the *TFEB* gene on locus 6p21. Translocation carcinoma generally arises in children and young adults, with increasing reports in patients older than 40 years. The prevalence of translocation carcinoma in adults has been estimated at 1%. In general, translocation carcinoma presents at a higher stage than clear cell RCC, with a high incidence of metastasis. The prognosis of patients with Xp11.2 RCC remains unclear. Early and smaller series reported an indolent course despite the often advanced stage at presentation. Recent series have reported a poorer prognosis for adult patients.[30]

Renal medullary carcinoma is a rare aggressive type of RCC associated almost exclusively with the sickle cell trait. This tumor is considered a more aggressive variant of collecting duct carcinoma, occurs in young patients, frequently presents with metastasis, and is associated with a very poor prognosis (mean duration of life after diagnosis of 19 weeks). The consistent loss of expression of INI1 protein in this tumor suggests that INI1 tumor suppressor gene plays a role in its pathogenesis.

OUTCOME ASSOCIATION ACROSS MAJOR HISTOLOGIC TYPES IN LOCALIZED RCC

Although distinct biologic differences among histologic types are accepted, proof of prognostic importance is required from evaluation of large cohort studies in which other associated clinical data and prognostic parameters are concurrently examined. Analysis of the data shows varying conclusions in the literature. A summary of these studies including more than 20,000 patients (**Table 7**) have focused on prognostic impact of histologic type based on the WHO 2004 classification. In an analysis of 588 patients from the earlier single-institution studies, Moch and colleagues[31] showed a better outcome for chromophobe carcinoma compared with clear cell RCC, but no difference between papillary and chromophobe RCC, and no statistical difference among the three groups. Subsequently, Amin and colleagues[25] examined 377 patients and showed that histologic type was associated with 5-year cancer-specific survival rates, which was significant on univariate analysis but not multivariate analysis. The limitation in these studies was the case size, which although numbering several hundred, remained statistically insufficiently powered to allow demonstration of outcome on multivariate analysis.

Subsequent studies analyzed histologic type against outcome using larger case numbers derived from assessing data from multiple institutions. Patard and colleagues[32] analyzed more than 4000 patients from eight institutions across Europe, and the United States. The distribution of types showed a higher proportion of clear cell compared with papillary and chromophobe RCC, and showed that histologic type was a significant predictor of outcome on univariate analysis but not on multivariate analysis. In another multi-institution study (from Iceland), Gudbjartsson and colleagues[33] examined 629 patients with a similarly high proportion of clear cell RCC compared with papillary and chromophobe RCC. The findings showed significant 5-year disease-specific survivals on univariate analysis but not on multivariate analysis.

In large single-institution studies (from Memorial Sloan-Kettering Cancer Center and Mayo Clinic), in which total case numbers exceeded those published in other earlier single-institution studies, outcome significance of RCC type was different. Teloken and colleagues,[34] reporting on 1863 patients from Memorial Sloan-Kettering Cancer Center (expanding on the cohort reported earlier by Beck and coauthors[35]), where histologic types were distributed as 72% clear cell, 17% papillary, and 12% chromophobe RCC, showed significant

Table 7
Series evaluating types of RCC with prognosis

Author	Case Size	M/S	Clear Cell RCC %	Clear Cell RCC 5-y DSS (%)	Papillary RCC %	Papillary RCC 5-y DSS (%)	Chromophobe RCC %	Chromophobe RCC 5-y DSS (%)	Univariate Analysis	Significance in Multivariate Analysis
Moch et al,[31] 2000	487	S	83	50	11	56	5	78	Yes	No
Amin et al,[25] 2002	405	S	63	70	5.9	88	5.7	94	Yes	No
Patard et al,[32] 2005	4063	M	87.7	73.2	9.7	79.4	2.5	87.9	Yes	No
Gudbjartsson et al,[33] 2005	629	M	88.7	54.9	8.4	66.5	2.1	84.6	Yes	No
Teloken et al,[34] 2009	1863	S	72	86	17	92	12	95	Yes	Yes
Leibovich et al,[36] 2010	3062	S	80.5	71	14.3	91	5.2	88	Yes	Yes
Capitanio et al,[38] 2009	11618	M	92.2	62	6.2	85.9	1.6	99.5	Yes	No

Abbreviations: DSS, disease-specific survival; M, multi-institution; S, single institution.

differences in 5-year disease-specific survival according to RCC type, with chromophobe and papillary RCC significantly associated with better outcome on multivariate analysis. Similarly, in the studies from the Mayo Clinic, Leibovich and colleagues[36] assessed histologic type and its correlation with survival as an extension of an earlier study from the Mayo Clinic by Cheville and colleagues.[37] In an evaluation of 3062 patients, they found a significant difference in cancer-specific survival between patients with clear cell RCC and the other histologic types; however, no significant difference was seen in outcome between patients with papillary and chromophobe types. Clear cell RCC remained a significant predictor of metastasis and cancer-specific death on multivariate analysis (when compared with stage, grade, tumor necrosis, and sarcomatoid differentiation).

In a more recent study by Capitanio and colleagues,[38] Surveillance, Epidemiology and End Results (SEER) data from nine American RCC cancer registries, totaling 11,618 cases, were examined to determine importance of histologic type in RCC survival. Histologic type stratified risk of cancer-specific mortality on univariate analysis and was an independent predictor of cancer-specific mortality. The significance, however, was lower than that for other variables (including age, year of surgery, TNM stage, and Fuhrman grade).

In summary, all five studies show that histologic type is important on univariate analysis and that clear cell RCC compared with papillary and chromophobe types predicts for higher stage and Fuhrman nuclear grade. In three of the five studies, an association of type with outcome is retained on multivariate analysis (when other key prognostic parameters are factored into the analysis). The confidence placed in the prognostic value of histologic type is evident by the use of histologic type in a prognostic nomogram (Kattan and colleagues[39]) at Memorial Sloan-Kettering Cancer Center, and as the basis for a postoperative surveillance program at the Mayo Clinic.[40]

The two reports in which histologic type retains strong significance above other prognostic variables are single-institution series (Mayo Clinic and Memorial Sloan-Kettering Cancer Center), wherein a single uropathologist or team of uropathologists working together evaluated every case and classified them in a predictably more standardized fashion. This practice is significantly different from that of other multi-institution studies that lacked central review.[32,33,38] The smaller cohort size in earlier reports (also from single institutions) resulted in a sample size in some categories that was insufficient to allow true statistical significance to be tested.[25,31]

The extent that centralized pathology review is important in the classification of RCC is shown in a study by Ficarra and colleagues,[41] in which rereview by a single uropathologist blinded to the original diagnosis showed only moderate concordance in cases diagnosed pre-1997, even though substantial concordance was achieved in the cases diagnosed after 1997. The lower concordance was because pathologists pre-1997 tended to lump all tumors with clear cell features into the clear cell category, even though some were papillary and chromophobe. Only after misclassification was corrected through centralized review did histologic type stratify cancer outcome. The much higher proportion of clear cell type in the multi-institution studies (87.7%–92.2%) compared with the Mayo Clinic and Memorial Sloan-Kettering Cancer Center series (80.5% and 72%) indicates a difference in histologic type assignment.

One may argue that academic center experience, in which highly experienced uropathologists perform RCC classification, is different from the experience in the community, where diagnosis is rendered by general pathologists. Pathologists' ability to accurately classify often depends on their experience and familiarity with a classification. In addition, special techniques such as immunohistochemistry offer useful tools for confirmation of RCC type, and are increasingly being used, suggesting that pathologists' assignment of RCC histologic type today may be more reliable than in the past.

In conclusion, the independent prognostic value of type is not widely accepted because of different results in series with varying study designs. Even though independent prognostic value may be debated, different histologic types are important to recognize for their different pathologic and clinical features, including predilections for different metastatic sites, stage associations, and likelihood for multicentricity. Underlying these differences are different molecular pathways. The differences based on histologic type already are used as rational methods for surveillance and adjuvant therapy while studies to resolve this debate continue.

DOES HISTOLOGIC TYPE INFLUENCE OUTCOME IN METASTATIC RCC?

The biologic differences in RCC types suggest that histologic type has prognostic and predictive potential also in metastatic RCC. In most studies, metastatic papillary and chromophobe RCC seem to have a worse prognosis than clear cell

RCC. In a series of metastatic RCC,[42] 64 patients (<10%) with non–clear cell type were found to be resistant to systemic cytokine and conventional therapy (particularly immunotherapy), with poor survival (overall survival of 9.4 months, with 29 months for those with chromophobe, 11 months for those with collecting duct, and 5.5 months for those with papillary RCC). In a trial on interleukin 2 (IL-2) that evaluated influence of histologic type on response to treatment, non–clear cell type showed a poor response to therapy.[43]

With the increasing use of targeted agents that inhibit angiogenic growth factors, the evaluation of histologic type is expected to play an important role as a rational method for determining therapy. Earlier trials restricted treatment to clear cell type; however, subsequent studies have shown response of metastatic papillary or chromophobe RCC to tyrosine kinase inhibitors (sorafenib or sunitinib).[44] Further studies are awaited to determine the most appropriate therapeutic strategy related to histologic type. Prospective controlled studies may enable data for predictive models to incorporate histologic type in nomograms for treatment of metastatic disease.

SIGNIFICANCE OF HISTOLOGIC TYPE: INCORPORATION INTO PROGNOSTIC ALGORITHMS IN RCC

Several prognostic algorithms or models[45] have been devised over the past decade to improve the accuracy of prognostic variables. These models combine prognostic variables in a weighted fashion into nomograms, as determined by their independent power on multivariate analysis in prior datasets. The various models include (1) the Memorial Sloan-Kettering Cancer Center localized RCC and conventional clear cell RCC monogram (2) the University of California Los Angeles Integrated Staging System, and (3) the Mayo Clinic stage, size, grade, and necrosis (SSIGN) score. These models use prognostic factors that may be tumor-related (stage, size, grade, histologic type, tumor necrosis, and sarcomatoid transformation), patient-related (systemic symptoms, performance status, weight loss, metastasis-free interval, history of prior nephrectomy), or derived from laboratory test results (elevated lactate dehydrogenase levels, hypercalcemia, anemia, elevated erythrocyte sedimentation rate, and thrombocytosis). To remain user-friendly and easily adapted to the clinical setting, the nomograms are limited to use of only variables of the most prognostic value. As support of its prognostic role, histologic type is used in a prognostic nomogram (Kattan and colleagues[39]) devised from one of these models. Its use has

been validated by external groups and found to be of greater value than three other similar models. The confidence placed in the prognostic value of histologic type is also evidenced by its use as the basis for a postoperative surveillance program at the Mayo Clinic.[40]

SUMMARY

Each histologic type of RCC shows differences in pathologic and clinical parameters, as well as prognostic relevance; however, the independent role of histologic type in outcome prediction remains contested. Most studies show relevance for outcome of each histologic type when correlated with survival on univariate analysis; however, only few studies are able to show differences in outcome when other key prognostic factors, such as stage and grade, are taken into account (using multivariate analysis). These studies with disparate results highlight the challenges to prove outcome relevance, such as the requirement for large cohort size to allow sufficient statistical strength and the importance of standardized pathology review, often missing in pooled multi-institution datasets. Despite the contested independent value of type for outcome prediction, separation of RCC into types is well accepted and can be substantiated on clinical, pathologic, molecular, and trends in outcome differences.

REFERENCES

1. Eble JN, Sauter G, Epstein JI, et al. Pathology and genetics of tumors of the urinary system and male genital organs. Lyon (France): IARC Press; 2004.
2. Kovacs G, Akhtar M, Beckwith BJ, et al. The Heidelberg classification of renal cell tumours. J Pathol 1997;183(2):131–3.
3. Storkel S, Eble JN, Adlakha K, et al. Classification of renal cell carcinoma: workgroup No. 1. Union Internationale Contre le Cancer (UICC) and the American Joint Committee on Cancer (AJCC). Cancer 1997; 80(5):987–9.
4. Thoenes W, Storkel S, Rumpelt HJ. Histopathology and classification of renal cell tumors (adenomas, oncocytomas and carcinomas). The basic cytological and histopathological elements and their use for diagnostics. Pathol Res Pract 1986;181(2): 125–43.
5. Edge SB, Byrd DR, Compton CC, et al, editors. AJCC cancer staging manual. 7th edition. New York (NY): Springer; 2010.
6. Adhya AK, Ahluwalia J, Varma N, et al. Abnormal chromatin clumping in leucocytes of Ph positive chronic myeloid leukemia cases: extending the

morphological spectrum. Indian J Pathol Microbiol 2008;51(4):548–50.

7. Frank I, Blute ML, Cheville JC, et al. Solid renal tumors: an analysis of pathological features related to tumor size. J Urol 2003;170(6 Pt 1):2217–20.

8. Thompson RH, Kurta JM, Kaag M, et al. Tumor size is associated with malignant potential in renal cell carcinoma cases. J Urol 2009;181(5):2033–6.

9. Paner GP, Amin MB, Alvarado-Cabrero I, et al. A novel tumor grading scheme for chromophobe renal cell carcinoma: prognostic utility and comparison with Fuhrman nuclear grade. Am J Surg Pathol 2010;34(9):1233–40.

10. Finley DS, Shuch B, Said JW, et al. The chromophobe tumor grading system is the preferred grading scheme for chromophobe renal cell carcinoma. J Urol 2011;186(6):2168–74.

11. Sika-Paotonu D, Bethwaite PB, McCredie MR, et al. Nucleolar grade but not Fuhrman grade is applicable to papillary renal cell carcinoma. Am J Surg Pathol 2006;30(9):1091–6.

12. Frank I, Blute ML, Cheville JC, et al. An outcome prediction model for patients with clear cell renal cell carcinoma treated with radical nephrectomy based on tumor stage, size, grade and necrosis: the SSIGN score. J Urol 2002;168(6):2395–400.

13. de Peralta-Venturina M, Moch H, Amin M, et al. Sarcomatoid differentiation in renal cell carcinoma: a study of 101 cases. Am J Surg Pathol 2001;25(3):275–84.

14. Grignon DJ, Eble JN, Bonsib SM, et al. Clear cell renal cell carcinoma. Lyon (France): IARC Press; 2004.

15. Lam JS, Leppert JT, Figlin RA, et al. Surveillance following radical or partial nephrectomy for renal cell carcinoma. Curr Urol Rep 2005;6(1):7–18.

16. Cindolo L, Patard JJ, Chiodini P, et al. Comparison of predictive accuracy of four prognostic models for nonmetastatic renal cell carcinoma after nephrectomy: a multicenter European study. Cancer 2005; 104(7):1362–71.

17. Tickoo SK, Reuter VE. Differential diagnosis of renal tumors with papillary architecture. Adv Anat Pathol 2011;18(2):120–32.

18. Thoenes W, Storkel S, Rumpelt HJ. Human chromophobe cell renal carcinoma. Virchows Arch B Cell Pathol Incl Mol Pathol 1985;48(3):207–17.

19. Klatte T, Remzi M, Zigeuner RE, et al. Development and external validation of a nomogram predicting disease specific survival after nephrectomy for papillary renal cell carcinoma. J Urol 2010;184(1): 53–8.

20. Lee JH, Choi JW, Kim YS. The value of histologic subtyping on outcomes of clear cell and papillary renal cell carcinomas: a meta-analysis. Urology 2010;76(4):889–94.

21. Przybycin CG, Cronin AM, Darvishian F, et al. Chromophobe renal cell carcinoma: a clinicopathologic study of 203 tumors in 200 patients with primary resection at a single institution. Am J Surg Pathol 2011;35(7):962–70.

22. Amin MB, Paner GP, Alvarado-Cabrero I, et al. Chromophobe renal cell carcinoma: histomorphologic characteristics and evaluation of conventional pathologic prognostic parameters in 145 cases. Am J Surg Pathol 2008;32(12):1822–34.

23. Wright JL, Risk MC, Hotaling J, et al. Effect of collecting duct histology on renal cell cancer outcome. J Urol 2009;182(6):2595–9.

24. Karakiewicz PI, Trinh QD, Rioux-Leclercq N, et al. Collecting duct renal cell carcinoma: a matched analysis of 41 cases. Eur Urol 2007;52(4):1140–5.

25. Amin MB, Tamboli P, Javidan J, et al. Prognostic impact of histologic subtyping of adult renal epithelial neoplasms: an experience of 405 cases. Am J Surg Pathol 2002;26(3):281–91.

26. Zisman A, Chao DH, Pantuck AJ, et al. Unclassified renal cell carcinoma: clinical features and prognostic impact of a new histological subtype. J Urol 2002;168(3):950–5.

27. Karakiewicz PI, Hutterer GC, Trinh QD, et al. Unclassified renal cell carcinoma: an analysis of 85 cases. BJU Int 2007;100(4):802–8.

28. Crispen PL, Tabian MR, Allmer C, et al. Unclassified renal cell carcinoma: impact on survival following nephrectomy. Urology 2010;76(3):580–6.

29. Suzigan S, Lopez-Beltran A, Montironi R, et al. Multilocular cystic renal cell carcinoma: a report of 45 cases of a kidney tumor of low malignant potential. Am J Clin Pathol 2006;125(2):217–22.

30. Komai Y, Fujiwara M, Fujii Y, et al. Adult Xp11 translocation renal cell carcinoma diagnosed by cytogenetics and immunohistochemistry. Clin Cancer Res 2009;15(4):1170–6.

31. Moch H, Gasser T, Amin MB, et al. Prognostic utility of the recently recommended histologic classification and revised TNM staging system of renal cell carcinoma: a Swiss experience with 588 tumors. Cancer 2000;89(3):604–14.

32. Patard JJ, Leray E, Rioux-Leclercq N, et al. Prognostic value of histologic subtypes in renal cell carcinoma: a multicenter experience. J Clin Oncol 2005; 23(12):2763–71.

33. Gudbjartsson T, Hardarson S, Petursdottir V, et al. Histological subtyping and nuclear grading of renal cell carcinoma and their implications for survival: a retrospective nation-wide study of 629 patients. Eur Urol 2005;48(4):593–600.

34. Teloken PE, Thompson RH, Tickoo SK, et al. Prognostic impact of histological subtype on surgically treated localized renal cell carcinoma. J Urol 2009; 182(5):2132–6.

35. Beck SD, Patel MI, Snyder ME, et al. Effect of papillary and chromophobe cell type on disease-free survival after nephrectomy for renal cell carcinoma. Ann Surg Oncol 2004;11(1):71–7.

36. Leibovich BC, Lohse CM, Crispen PL, et al. Histological subtype is an independent predictor of outcome for patients with renal cell carcinoma. J Urol 2010;183(4):1309–15.

37. Cheville JC, Lohse CM, Zincke H, et al. Comparisons of outcome and prognostic features among histologic subtypes of renal cell carcinoma. Am J Surg Pathol 2003;27(5):612–24.

38. Capitanio U, Cloutier V, Zini L, et al. A critical assessment of the prognostic value of clear cell, papillary and chromophobe histological subtypes in renal cell carcinoma: a population-based study. BJU Int 2009;103(11):1496–500.

39. Kattan MW, Reuter V, Motzer RJ, et al. A postoperative prognostic nomogram for renal cell carcinoma. J Urol 2001;166(1):63–7.

40. Siddiqui SA, Frank I, Cheville JC, et al. Postoperative surveillance for renal cell carcinoma: a multifactorial histological subtype specific protocol. BJU Int 2009; 104(6):778–85.

41. Ficarra V, Martignoni G, Galfano A, et al. Prognostic role of the histologic subtypes of renal cell carcinoma after slide revision. Eur Urol 2006;50(4):786–93 [discussion: 793–4].

42. Motzer RJ, Bacik J, Mariani T, et al. Treatment outcome and survival associated with metastatic renal cell carcinoma of non-clear-cell histology. J Clin Oncol 2002;20(9):2376–81.

43. Upton MP, Parker RA, Youmans A, et al. Histologic predictors of renal cell carcinoma response to interleukin-2-based therapy. J Immunother 2005; 28(5):488–95.

44. Sun M, Lughezzani G, Perrotte P, et al. Treatment of metastatic renal cell carcinoma. Nature reviews. Urology 2010;7(6):327–38.

45. Galfano A, Novara G, Iafrate M, et al. Mathematical models for prognostic prediction in patients with renal cell carcinoma. Urol Int 2008;80(2):113–23.

46. Zucchi A, Novara G, Costantini E, et al. Prognostic factors in a large multi-institutional series of papillary renal cell carcinoma. BJU Int, in press.

47. Sukov WR, Lohse CM, Leibovich BC, et al. Clinical and pathological features associated with prognosis in patients with papillary renal cell carcinoma. J Urol 2012;187(1):54–9.

48. Klatte T, Han KR, Said JW, et al. Pathobiology and prognosis of chromophobe renal cell carcinoma. Urol Oncol 2008;26(6):604–9.

49. Volpe A, Novara G, Antonelli A, et al. Chromophobe renal cell carcinoma (RCC): oncological outcomes and prognostic factors in a large multicentre series. BJU Int, in press.

50. Lee WK, Byun SS, Kim HH, et al. Characteristics and prognosis of chromophobe non-metastatic renal cell carcinoma: a multicenter study. Int J Urol 2010; 17(11):898–904.

51. Tokuda N, Naito S, Matsuzaki O, et al. Collecting duct (Bellini duct) renal cell carcinoma: a nationwide survey in Japan. J Urol 2006;176(1):40–3 [discussion: 43].

The Surgical Approach to Multifocal Renal Cancers: Hereditary Syndromes, Ipsilateral Multifocality, and Bilateral Tumors

Brian Shuch, MD[a], Eric A. Singer, MD, MA[a],
Gennady Bratslavsky, MD[a,b],*

KEYWORDS

- Renal cell carcinoma • Bilateral kidney cancer
- Multifocal kidney cancer • Hereditary kidney cancer

The management of a localized renal cell carcinoma (RCC) continues to evolve with fewer radical surgeries and increase in nephron preservation.[1] Reasons for this include recognition of the importance of renal preservation, the emergence of both partial nephrectomy and adrenal sparing, and a more minimally invasive surgical approach. The approach to a sporadic renal mass smaller than 7 cm can provide treatment dilemmas to clinicians, as the American Urologic Association suggests several acceptable management options for patients.[2]

Dealing with patients with bilateral, multifocal, kidney cancer adds an additional layer of complexity. Clinicians should be familiar with these entities, as they will undoubtedly come across patients with multifocal bilateral renal masses. With this patient population, the clinician should consider a variety of factors, including hereditary predisposition, need to stage bilateral operations, which kidney to operate on first, prolonged ischemic times, how to define recurrence, how to manage recurrence in a previously operated renal unit, and the possibility of progression to end-stage renal failure.

DEFINITIONS OF MULTIFOCALITY AND BILATERALITY

Sporadic, unilateral renal tumors account for most patients with kidney cancer; however, patients with multiple renal masses are not uncommon, and clinicians who specialize in RCC will eventually be faced with the management of these patients.[3] Multifocality in kidney cancer refers to having more than one renal tumor, which can further be divided into whether the additional tumors are ipsilateral or bilateral. Bilateral tumors refer to lesions on both kidneys and they can present in a synchronous manner (at the same time) or a metachronous fashion (at different times). Multifocality and bilaterality are entities frequently seen together; bilateral renal involvement is observed in 90% of those with multifocal disease and the converse is true that more than half of patients with bilateral tumors have multifocal RCC.[3–5]

Several series have found that the incidence of bilateral, synchronous renal masses is approximately 2% of individuals who present with renal masses[4,6]; however, even among patients who

[a] Urologic Oncology Branch, National Cancer Institute, National Institutes of Health, Building 10, CRC, Room 1-5940, Bethesda, MD 20892, USA
[b] Department of Urology, SUNY Upstate Medical University, 750 East Adams Street, Syracuse, NY 13210, USA
* Corresponding author. Department of Urology, SUNY Upstate Medical University, 750 East Adams Street, Syracuse, NY 13210.
E-mail address: bratslag@upstate.edu

Urol Clin N Am 39 (2012) 133–148
doi:10.1016/j.ucl.2012.01.006
0094-0143/12/$ – see front matter © 2012 Elsevier Inc. All rights reserved.

had a sporadic, solitary renal mass, contralateral metachronous renal masses occur in about 1% to 2% of patients.[7–9] It is important to recognize that multifocal tumors have been found in as many as 25% of patients in some studies, and many multifocal RCCs will be bilateral.[5,10] Patients also may present with a unilateral multifocal tumor complicating surgical planning and possibly causing some urologists to shy away from a partial nephrectomy. These patients, however, are likely the most in need of nephron-sparing surgery, as they would have a high propensity to form additional tumors in the contralateral kidney.

The estimated incidence of multifocality widely varies based on how the series was performed. Some series estimate multifocality by preoperative imaging, yet cross-sectional imaging studies frequently miss these small satellite lesions in more than 75% of cases.[11] Other series include unknown lesions seen at the time of surgery. Based on these different definitions, the incidence is reported to be between 3% and 11%.[12–14] Other reports based on pathologic examination demonstrate multifocality to be as high as 25% of radical nephrectomy specimens based on the presence of microscopic satellite tumors.[10,15,16] Although papillary RCC more commonly presents with multifocality, all histologic subtypes can have satellite tumors.[8,9,17]

DESCRIPTION OF HEREDITARY RENAL SYNDROME PHENOTYPES

Hereditary kidney cancer is believed to represent 1% to 4% of RCC cases. Of these patients, some may fit into well-characterized hereditary kidney cancer syndromes, whereas many more patients with RCC may have a genetic component that is not fully recognized or understood. Because of our current poor understanding of genetics and cancer susceptibility genes, the 1% to 4% estimate may be a gross underestimation. A generational study from Iceland (dating back 11 centuries) has aggregated nearly 60% of RCC to specific families. These data suggest that unknown germline mutations may account for a large number of these apparently sporadic cases of kidney cancer.[18] The complexity of inherited susceptibility loci associated with RCC continues to be elucidated by genome-wide association studies.[19,20]

During the past 3 decades, more than a half-dozen hereditary cancer conditions have been described and linked to specific germline mutations. Alterations for these syndromes generally occur in tumor suppressor genes, however proto-oncogene alterations can be responsible

as well. Because additional events are likely necessary for renal tumorigenesis, these syndromes have different penetrance of renal malignancy. Although these conditions often share a common manifestation of bilateral, multifocal kidney tumors, they differ in the tumor histology, coexistence with renal cysts, and additional clinical features. For patients without a previously diagnosed syndrome, an astute clinician with knowledge of these conditions may be the key to a successful diagnosis. Particular attention must focus on patients' past medical history, including a thorough review of systems. A thorough family medical history must detail the health of both maternal and paternal family members. Although most patients are diagnosed based on the presentation and a known family history, new diagnosis is not uncommon, because some patients are unaware of family history, are adopted, or there is the possibility of a de novo mutation. If a clinician is going to be involved in the care of these patients, an awareness of the genetic basis and associated features of these syndromes is necessary to appropriately recognize who may benefit from genetic counseling.

Von Hippel-Lindau

Von Hippel-Lindau (VHL) is an autosomal dominant syndrome with an incidence of 1:35,000 individuals. The syndrome is characterized by the development of clear-cell RCC in addition to multiple tumor types, including retinal angiomas, spinal and cerebellar hemangioblastomas, pancreatic cysts and neuroendocrine tumors, pheochromocytomas, and epididymal cystadenomas. Linkage analyses from kindred with affected individuals determined the gene for VHL to be located at 3p.[21] Later work located the VHL gene to 3p25.1 and determined it behaved like a classic tumor suppressor gene.[22,23]

Patients with VHL are prone to the development of both renal cysts and clear-cell renal tumors. Approximately 25% to 60% of patients with VHL develop RCC and, when it occurs, it generally is bilateral and multifocal.[24] Before the current screening recommendations, approximately a third of patients with VHL died from metastatic kidney cancer.[25] With proper screening, patients at risk are identified when the lesions are small and treatment can prevent the development of metastatic disease.

Birt-Hogg-Dube

Birt-Hogg-Dube (BHD) is a hereditary cancer syndrome first discovered in the dermatologic literature when 3 physicians described a kindred of 70 patients with multiple fibrofolliculomas associated with trichodiscomas and acrochordons.[26] Later, patients with BHD were found to have bilateral, multifocal RCC and pneumothoraces that were determined to be part of the syndrome.[27,28] Linkage analysis of kindreds with BHD found the gene was located on 17p11.2.[29] The gene for BHD was determined to be *FLCN,* which behaves like a classic tumor suppressor syndrome and is passed in an autosomal dominant fashion.[30]

BHD is believed to be fairly rare, with an incidence estimated to be approximately 1:200,000. When evaluating these patients, a history of a pneumothorax or a thorough dermatologic evaluation may be a clue to the diagnosis. On imaging, renal cysts may occur with BHD, but when present, they are generally simple, unlike mixed lesions in VHL. Approximately 18% of patients with BHD develop renal tumors, and when they occur, they are generally multifocal and bilateral.[31] Tumors can be multiple histologies, with hybrid oncocytic and chromophobe renal tumors the most common (50% and 35%, respectively).[32] Clear-cell renal tumors associated with BHD are rare, but when they occur, they can be quite aggressive.[33]

Hereditary Leiomyomatosis and Renal Cell Cancer

Hereditary leiomyomatosis and renal cell cancer (HLRCC) is an autosomal dominant syndrome first recognized more than 50 years ago as being responsible for familial, cutaneous leiomyomas.[34] Later an association with uterine fibroids and RCC was identified.[35–37] Familial linkage analysis identified the chromosomal region to 1p42.3–43 and later determined the responsible gene was fumarate hydratase, *FH.*[35,38,39] This key enzyme is responsible for conversion of fumarate to malate in the Kreb's cycle, and loss of the remaining wild-type copy leads to anaerobic respiration.

The renal tumors associated with HLRCC were first described to be papillary type II.[40] Later reports in a larger subset of renal tumors demonstrated that these tumors may have other patterns besides a papillary configuration, but the unifying hallmark is the large eosinophilic nucleolus with a clear perinucleolar halo.[41] Although most patients with hereditary kidney cancer syndromes frequently have bilateral, multifocal kidney tumors, the early experience with HLRCC did not show this phenotype, likely because of the aggressive nature of this disease.[41] The first clinical series demonstrated that approximately half of patients presented with nodal or disseminated disease,

even in the presence of small T1 renal masses.[42] With early identification and screening, however, treatment before spread has now demonstrated the bilateral and multifocal nature of the disease.

Hereditary Papillary Renal Cell Carcinoma

Hereditary papillary renal cell carcinoma (HPRC) was first recognized almost 20 years ago in a family with 3 generations of papillary RCC that did not appear linked to chromosome 3p.[43] Besides the occurrence of kidney cancer, no other clinical manifestations have been found. The gene was linked to 7q31 and the gene, *MET,* was found to be an important receptor tyrosine kinase.[44] Trisomy 7 is common in HPRC and it preferentially amplifies the mutant copy.[45] Unlike the other hereditary kidney cancer syndromes associated with germline mutations, *MET* is a proto-oncogene.[44]

HPRC is a rare syndrome with fewer than 20 families described with this entity. It is passed in an autosomal dominant fashion and is highly penetrant. Nearly 70% of carriers develop renal tumors; however, the mean age of tumor occurrence is nearly 50, older than observed with the other hereditary syndromes.

A recent trial performed at the National Cancer Institute (NCI) evaluating small molecules targeting MET receptors has shown excellent tumor response in patients with HPRC.[46] Such targeted approaches (presently being tested in other hereditary renal cancers) may in the future delay the need for surgical intervention or perhaps avoid a need for surgery altogether.

Succinate Dehydrogenase B Deficiency

Several syndromes are associated with hereditary causes of pheochromocytoma and paraganglioma. Many of these patients have been found with germline mutations in subunits of the succinate dehydrogenase (SDH) enzyme, an inner mitochondrial membrane enzyme critical to both the Kreb's cycle and the electron transport chain. In 2001, the *SDHB* gene was found mutated in families with hereditary pheochromocytoma and paraganglioma, and this gene is passed in an autosomal dominant fashion.[47] Several years later, a family with a known *SDHB* mutation was found to contain 2 individuals with early-onset RCC.[48] Screening of RCC families without a known mutation has demonstrated that nearly 5% have *SDHB* mutations.[49] Patients with *SDHB* can present with early-onset and bilateral renal tumors. The distinctive morphology of *SDHB* renal tumors is still being elucidated; however, a recent report mentions these tumors contained indistinct cell borders, cytoplasmic inclusions, and eosinophilic cytoplasm.[50]

Tuberous Sclerosis 1 and 2

Tuberous sclerosis complex (TSC) is an autosomal dominant condition that is characterized by tumors in the brain, skin, and kidney. Germline mutations can be found in 2 related genes, TSC1 and TSC2, both of which act like classic tumor suppressor genes. TSC1 and TSC2 encode for hamartin (located on 9q34) and tuberin (located on 16p13.3), respectively.[51,52] Renal manifestations occur early and are highly penetrant. These features include angiomyolipomas, cysts, and clear-cell RCC. Patients can progress to renal failure, possibly attributable to these lesions or to other factors currently poorly understood.[53] Although considered benign, angiomyolipomas can grow and cause significant morbidity related to pain and risk of hemorrhage. TSC-related clear-cell RCC can behave quite aggressively, with many patients dying from their disease.[54] Genetic analysis of these renal tumors demonstrates that loss of 3p and VHL mutations are uncommon with these tumors.[55]

Familial Renal Oncocytoma/Bilateral Multifocal Oncocytoma

Oncocytomas are benign tumors that account for roughly 10% of enhancing renal masses. Oncocytomas are bilateral or multifocal in 5% and 13% of cases, respectively.[56,57] Patients with multifocal renal lesions with a known history of oncocytoma (either in the setting of a synchronous, contralateral oncocytoma or a new metachronous tumor) demonstrate pathologic concordance in more than 70% of cases.[58,59] The pathologic term, oncocytomatosis (later called oncocytosis), has been used to describe the constellation of findings including multiple microscopic, oncocytic nodules and oncocytic changes in the non-neoplastic tubules.[60] For unclear reasons, these patients appear to have renal insufficiency, with many progressing to end-stage renal disease.[61,62] A familial form has been named familial renal oncocytoma (FRO) and affected individuals develop bilateral and multifocal oncocytomas.[63] The gene for FRO has not been described, but research efforts are currently ongoing.

Bilateral/Multifocal and Familial Renal Cancer of Unknown Etiology

Patients with a first-degree or second-degree relative with kidney cancer are considered to have familial renal cancer (FRC). Even after genetic counseling, many patients will not have an identifiable gene mutation; however, this does not rule out a genetic component involved in their familial predisposition. The number of known germline cancer syndromes continues to rise and, with time, many of these families could have a predisposing genetic factor identified. Many patients with FRC will present with bilateral and multifocal RCC.

The management of these patients is often dependent on the number of lesions and the size of the largest lesion. In most instances, these patients are recommended to undergo a percutaneous biopsy of the largest or most accessible lesion (occasionally more than one). This often allows for preoperative planning, a possible need for a resection of a wider margin or lymph node dissection, or additional imaging studies. In some instances, percutaneous biopsy of these patients allows for avoidance of surgical intervention if bilateral multifocal oncocytomas are diagnosed. Should surgery be planned, these patients are treated with partial nephrectomy whenever possible, as they can be prone to future development of new renal lesions. Enucleation can also be performed with these patients, especially in those with multifocal tumors, as they are likely to develop de novo lesions. Observation of small renal lesions until the largest lesion measures 3 cm may also be a feasible option.

PRINCIPLES AND GOALS OF SURGICAL MANAGEMENT

For patients with sporadic, solitary renal tumors, the goal of therapy is cancer cure while maximizing renal function. With sporadic patients, a single surgery is likely to be sufficient, with surveillance most commonly aimed at identification of cancer dissemination. In the sporadic population, RCC usually presents in patients in their 60s, and although not ideal, a radiographically normal-appearing contralateral kidney gives the clinician the option of sacrificing an affected kidney in the setting of a large tumor requiring a complex partial nephrectomy. For patients with bilateral, multifocal, and hereditary renal tumors, the goal of therapy is much different. These patients generally present with tumors at a younger age and the clinician has to be forward thinking, not just worrying about the current tumors, but what may develop in the future. The goal of therapy in this population is to prevent cancer dissemination, while maximizing renal function, limiting the number of renal surgeries, and minimizing the amount of surgical morbidity when possible.

Historical Management

Traditional management of synchronous, bilateral renal masses included bilateral radical nephrectomy to prevent dissemination and death from kidney cancer and dialysis.[64] With this approach, patients could receive either concomitant or delayed renal transplantation.[65–67] For patients with VHL disease, this was a common approach in some centers.[68–70] Fortunately, this approach is no longer widely accepted with the advent and increasing acceptance of partial nephrectomy.

Preservation of Renal Function

In patients with bilateral, multifocal, and hereditary kidney tumors, preservation of renal function is one of the most important aspects of therapy. Whenever feasible, a partial nephrectomy should be considered if there is potential to avoid dialysis. Because of the significant cardiovascular morbidity and mortality associated with renal replacement therapy, the overall risk on dialysis is often greater than the risk from renal malignancy. The 5-year overall survival on dialysis of 33% is far worse than the survival for nearly all stages of localized disease.[71] Although survival on dialysis is poor in general, in patients with RCC, survival may actually be worse.[72] Although patients with RCC placed on dialysis may be transplant candidates, many will die waiting for an organ because of the shortage of available donors and the 2-year cancer-free interval suggested by the American Society of Transplantation.[71,73,74]

WORKUP AND MANAGEMENT

Patients presenting with bilateral, multifocal, and possibly hereditary renal tumors present management dilemmas. Decisions on timing of genetic testing, role of biopsy, likelihood of pathologic concordance, order of surgery, sequence of tumor removal, optimal methods of nephron preservation, and surveillance for de novo lesions are unique to this patient population. Management of these patients is largely based on more than 20 years of NCI experience with excellent oncologic outcomes. We discuss our experience on the workup and management of these patients.

Preoperative Testing: Percutaneous Biopsy, Renogram

We suggest an algorithm for the workup and management of patients with bilateral, multifocal, and known or suspected hereditary syndromes (**Fig. 1**). For those without a known condition, genetic testing can be very helpful if a syndrome is identified. When there is no preliminary evidence of a hereditary syndrome, preoperative biopsy of the largest lesion(s) often guides histology-directed genetic testing. This strategy could also reduce the expense associated with genetic counseling by narrowing down the candidate syndromes.

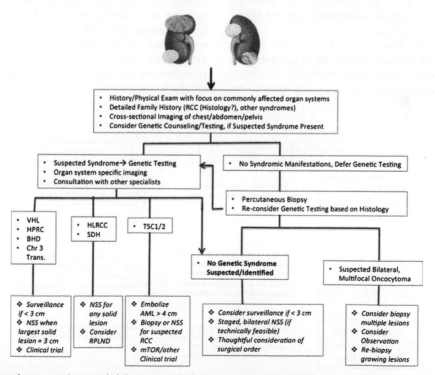

Fig. 1. Approach to a patient with bilateral, multifocal renal tumors or FRC.

Nuclear scintigraphy with a Mag-3 renogram is useful for preoperative imaging in patients with bilateral renal tumors. This test serves as a baseline to better delineate split renal function. Information gained from the nuclear scan may help with surgical planning or alter surgical approach. For a staged approach, it is useful to assess how the prior renal unit has recovered from the surgery, as resection of dozens of tumors may have to be performed in a single setting.[75] In the setting of a large decrease in renal function, delaying surgery to allow additional recovery may be warranted. If the kidney demonstrates very poor function (<15% split function), functionally the patient is considered to have a solitary kidney. In this situation, the surgeons may consider an open surgical approach over laparoscopic technique if they feel it will minimize total ischemia or warm ischemia time.

For synchronous, bilateral renal tumors that require intervention, the timing of surgery is open to debate. Three main surgical options exist for patients with synchronous, bilateral renal masses that require intervention, and include (1) concomitant, bilateral partial nephrectomy, (2) staged partial nephrectomy with the larger/more complex side first, and (3) staged partial nephrectomy with the smaller/less complex side first. Although some centers feel comfortable performing concomitant renal surgery, many surgeons prefer a staged approach because of concerns for potential complications, such as postoperative renal failure from bilateral renal surgery.

Deciding on the approach deserves much thought in each unique case, as arguments can be made for all 3 circumstances (**Fig. 2**). The bilateral renal surgery approach allows surgery to be performed in a single setting; however, if problems occur on the first side there is a risk that the second side would need to be aborted. Performing a bilateral laparoscopic partial nephrectomy is difficult owing to patient positioning changes and is often not feasible. Should the concomitant, bilateral approach be chosen it often requires a midline/chevron incision, but may result in having a need to manage bilateral complications simultaneously. For a staged approach in the absence of metastatic disease, it may be prudent to operate on the larger tumor first, as it may pose a greater threat for dissemination. In the setting of surgeries that have different complexities, it may be preferable to do the less complex side first in case the more challenging tumor necessitates a radical nephrectomy. If done in the opposite order and a radical nephrectomy was required, prolonged clamping of a solitary kidney could place the patient at risk for significant renal complications. At the NCI, the typical approach is via staged procedures performed through the flank retroperitoneal approaches.

Partial Nephrectomy, the "3-cm Rule," and Enucleation

Although surgical site recurrence rates are low and typically associated with grossly positive surgical margins at the time of nephron-sparing surgery (NSS), the management of locally recurrent disease or metachronous multifocal disease in the ipsilateral renal unit is challenging.[76] The NCI experience of managing familial renal cancer syndromes, such as VHL, HPRC, and BHD, provides unique insight into the management of locally recurrent RCC.[77]

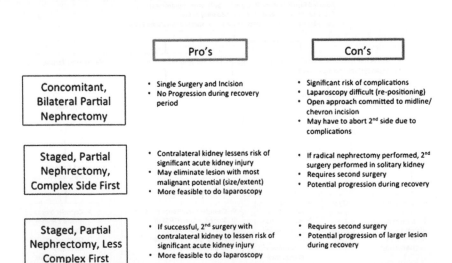

	Pro's	Con's
Concomitant, Bilateral Partial Nephrectomy	• Single Surgery and Incision • No Progression during recovery period	• Significant risk of complications • Laparoscopy difficult (re-positioning) • Open approach committed to midline/chevron incision • May have to abort 2nd side due to complications
Staged, Partial Nephrectomy, Complex Side First	• Contralateral kidney lessens risk of significant acute kidney injury • May eliminate lesion with most malignant potential (size/extent) • More feasible to do laparoscopy	• If radical nephrectomy performed, 2nd surgery performed in solitary kidney • Requires second surgery • Potential progression during recovery
Staged, Partial Nephrectomy, Less Complex First	• If successful, 2nd surgery with contralateral kidney to lessen risk of significant acute kidney injury • More feasible to do laparoscopy	• Requires second surgery • Potential progression of larger lesion during recovery

Fig. 2. Surgical approaches to bilateral, synchronous renal masses.

To preserve renal function, maximize the time interval between repeat partial nephrectomies, and minimize the risk of metastasis, the NCI uses the "3-cm rule" as a size threshold for surgical decision making. When the largest solid tumor in a given kidney measures 3 cm in diameter, NSS is recommended via enucleation of all detectable solid lesions within that renal unit.[78,79] The size of the negative margin needed to maintain oncologic efficacy is small and the attainment of wide margins comes directly at the cost of preserved renal parenchyma.[80]

Experience with enucleative surgery in patients with hereditary RCC has been applied to the management of sporadic RCC. Enucleative surgery for well-encapsulated masses, in which no margin of normal parenchyma is excised, has been reported for sporadic tumors. Enucleation did not seem to hamper survival outcomes when compared with partial nephrectomys in which a margin is taken.[81–83] This approach may be especially useful in patients with significant preoperative renal insufficiency or multifocal disease.

It should be noted, however, that the 3-cm rule was initially developed in patients with VHL and then applied to patients with HPRC and BHD. Patients with HLRCC, which is associated with papillary type 2 tumors that are known for their early metastatic potential, are never observed. Once a solid renal tumor is detected in patients with HLRCC, the surgical extirpation is recommended and includes a margin of normal parenchyma. Because of a high predilection of lymphatic spread of HLRCC tumors, a retroperitoneal lymphadenectomy is often performed as well.[42] Because of the aggressive nature of SDH renal tumors and altered metabolism similar to HLRCC, the patients with SDHB and renal tumors are treated in a fashion similar to patients with HLRCC.

The 3-cm rule requires a careful balance between oncologic efficacy and renal preservation. Although there have been significant advances in the use of systemic targeted therapies to treat locally advanced and metastatic RCC, these agents are not considered curative and are associated with significant toxicities. This fact highlights the importance of timely and effective surgical management for bilateral multifocal tumors or local recurrences.[84]

TECHNICAL CONSIDERATIONS

An operation on patients with bilateral, multifocal, and hereditary kidney cancer has unique technical aspects that differ from that of sporadic renal masses. The likelihood of requiring repeat renal surgeries is high and therefore the surgeon must be cognizant of maximizing renal function while minimizing unnecessary steps that could hinder future surgical approaches. Such steps may limit unnecessary morbidity of future operations that are often fraught with complications. Although none of these techniques discussed have been tested in a randomized fashion, we have used them for years and believe that these small, technical considerations are useful in this patient population.

Minimally Invasive Techniques

A minimally invasive partial nephrectomy in the setting of multifocal renal masses is challenging but can be performed in experienced hands. Both laparoscopic and robotic approaches have been described.[85–87] In the setting of synchronous tumors, surgery for a solitary lesion can be performed similar to sporadic cases, with the exception that clamp time should be minimized or avoided if possible. For those with multifocal, ipsilateral lesions, it is useful to consider performing the less complex lesions initially with an off-clamp approach.[85] The renal hilum should be accessible for clamping if excessive bleeding ensues.

In the population with hereditary RCC, prior ipsilateral, retroperitoneal surgery is common owing to prior renal and adrenal surgeries. A laparoscopic partial nephrectomy approach may be feasible; however, patients must understand the risk of open conversion. Boris and colleagues[88] reviewed the NCI experience with laparoscopic surgery after prior ipsilateral kidney/adrenal surgeries. In this cohort, roughly a quarter of patients required open conversion. Although this series has encouraging outcomes, proper patient selection cannot be overemphasized.

Retroperitoneal Flank Approach

For an open partial nephrectomy, multiple surgical incisions can be chosen to access the kidney, including midline, chevron, thoracoabdominal, and flank/retroperitoneal approaches. Our preference is to perform surgery via a retroperitoneal approach when possible via a mini-flank incision off the tip of the 11th rib. A major advantage of keeping the case retroperitoneal is avoiding the peritoneal cavity and limiting adjacent organ adherence to the kidney and renal hilum. Dissection of these organs off the kidney can be fraught with complications.[89,90] An additional advantage of staying retroperitoneal is to contain postoperative fluid collections to a confined space. Keeping a hematoma or urine leak in this confined space may prevent bowel dysfunction and facilitate easier fluid removal with a postoperative drain.

Preservation of Gerota Fascia

Accessing the kidney through Gerota fascia for a partial nephrectomy requires limited planning with sporadic renal tumors. The surgeon simply opens the fascia and dissects the perinephric fat off the kidney to inspect the mass of interest and to determine if there are any satellite lesions. Removal of the Gerota fascia and perinephric fat is often performed along with the specimen. In patients who have bilateral, multifocal, and hereditary renal tumors, this part of the surgery should be performed in a calculated fashion. There is abundant blood flow within Gerota fascia, much of it coming off the renal hilum and small collaterals off the kidney.[91] Haphazard dissection of the Gerota fascia off the kidney and renal hilum is likely to devascularize this structure. If the Gerota fascia and perinephric fat are left in place, completely devascularized fat necrosis can occur. Besides causing difficulty interpreting postoperative imaging, fat necrosis can lead to scarring of the Gerota fascia to the peritoneum. We attempt to open Gerota fascia in only one location to prevent devascularization.

Once the operation is completed, reapproximation of Gerota fascia will serve as a barrier between the peritoneum and the kidney, assist with hemostasis, and aid with the future reexplorations of retroperitoneum. For future operations, this protective barrier can serve to limit the fusion of retroperitoneal contents to the kidney. Limiting potential bowel and pancreatic adhesions to the kidney likely limits the risk of damaging these organs.

En Bloc Hilar Dissection

Minimizing dissection around the renal hilum limits scarring and facilitates future vascular control. Dissecting hilum en bloc has decreased our vascular complications rates and blood loss, as those have been quite common in our earlier experience.[89,90] For vascular control, we prefer to control the renal artery and vein en bloc with a Cosgrove vascular clamp. By minimizing hilar dissection and the skeletanization of the adventitia encasing the renal vessels, scarring of the renal hilum is decreased. Together these steps may facilitate easier vascular control in the future and limit the risk of major pedicle injuries.

Intraoperative Ultrasound

We recommend intraoperative ultrasound for all bilateral, multifocal partial nephrectomies to maximize tumor cleanout and avoid unnecessary ischemic time.[92–94] Depending on the operative approach, a handheld or laparoscopic ultrasound probe can be placed directly on the renal parenchyma for delineation of the renal anatomy and identification of all tumors. Some lesions that are too small to characterize on cross-sectional imaging may be better visualized on ultrasound and then removed if they are solid. For completely endophytic lesions, ultrasound can define the plan of dissection through the normal parenchyma directly down to the tumor.

Tumor Resection Planning

Removal of tumors under ischemia may allow better identification of the margin of the tumor by palpation of tissue turgor and visualization in a bloodless field[95]; however, this added benefit comes with a cost of ischemia and nephronal loss. Studies evaluating renal function have demonstrated that resection with no ischemia better preserves renal function than with ischemia.[96] Although it is believed that longer ischemic times lead to worse outcomes, the optimal duration of ischemia is unclear and may partly depend on nonmodifiable patient factors.[97,98] Despite this uncertainty, some groups suggest limiting warm and cold ischemic times to less than 20 and 35 minutes, respectively.[99]

For patients with multifocal and bilateral disease, the research involving ischemia during partial nephrectomy may be less relevant. Removal of multiple renal tumors with the renal hilum clamped could necessitate a prolonged ischemic time and lead to permanent renal dysfunction. Once the kidney is fully mobilized, surgical planning must focus on delineating the order of resection. We try to limit the potential ischemic time by planning to remove all exophytic lesions off clamp starting with the easiest lesion and then move to more difficult lesions. Extensive communication with the anesthesiologist is necessary to optimize fluid resuscitation. While off clamp, rather than rapidly progressing from one lesion to the next, greater emphasis is placed on minimizing bleeding and allowing the anesthesia team to catch up with losses. Near the end of the procedure, the more challenging endophytic and/or hilar lesions are attempted. Resection may be started off clamp and later converted to clamping, if needed. Once the tumor is removed and the patient is stable, early unclamping allows us to perform the renorrhaphy while minimizing ischemic time. With this approach, it is not uncommon to remove dozens of tumors with less than several minutes of ischemic time; patients should be aware that transfusions are commonly required.

Tumor Enucleation

Obtaining a margin while removing multiple kidney tumors in patients with multifocal disease would result in significant loss of renal parenchyma and is an impractical approach. First, because of the multifocal nature of the tumors, resecting normal parenchyma often identifies microscopic lesions not visible to a naked eye, cross-sectional imaging, or ultrasound. Second, each resection with a parenchymal margin could enter vital, irreplaceable, arterioles and lead to significant bleeding. Ligation of multiple vessels at the tumor base could lead to devitalization of a significant area of remaining parenchyma. In addition, performing such operations would require prolonged ischemic times and put the remaining parenchyma at risk.

Therefore, in patients with multifocal lesions, the tumor is resected by following the tumoral pseudocapsule. Such type of resection has been termed enucleative resection and is most useful especially in patients with multiple renal masses. An enucleative resection in this patient population allows for rapid tumor removal, avoidance of significant bleeding, and maximal renal preservation.[100] For small, sporadic tumors this approach has also demonstrated excellent oncologic outcome.[81]

Hemostasis

Removal of the tumors by enucleation off clamp may limit bleeding but requires identification of the correct plane throughout the resection. The surgeon should be prepared to encounter unexpected hemorrhage from the tumor base and be able to repair the resection defect rapidly, trying to avoid repeat clamping and unclamping of the renal hilum. The use of 2 suctions to maximize visualization during resection is recommended. Mini-clips can be applied if small vessels are identified before dividing or focal compression with a Kitner dissector on an open vessel may be required to decrease the risk bleeding. This can later be controlled with a dissolvable suture after tumor removal.

Venous bleeding is also common from the tumor base. Unnecessary suturing at the tumor base may compromise vascular supply to the surrounding normal parenchyma and should be avoided. Venous hemostasis can be controlled with manual compression using thrombin-soaked gel foam and a gauze sponge. While remaining off clamp, the surgeon has the luxury of waiting for bleeding to subside before moving on to the next lesion.

SPECIAL FOLLOW-UP CONCERNS: RECURRENCE VERSUS DE NOVO TUMOR DEVELOPMENT

In patients with sporadic renal tumors, a major goal of follow-up is aimed at early identification of distant disease. Although this is also true with those with bilateral, multifocal, and hereditary syndromes, the likelihood of new tumor development is much higher. Understanding the definition of recurrence and how to manage tumors when they occur is critical for any clinician taking care of this patient population.

Defining Local Recurrence

The concept of local recurrence in kidney cancer is difficult to define and may be present for several reasons. Tumor noted on postoperative surveillance imaging can be found because of incomplete resection of the primary tumor at the time of partial nephrectomy; growth of an adjacent, existing tumor; or development of de novo tumor. Unsuspected tumor multifocality has been identified in a quarter of patients undergoing partial nephrectomy, and individuals affected by familial renal cancer syndromes are known to develop bilateral multifocal disease.[10,15,16,101,102] The most common and still underappreciated cause of tumor recurrence is multifocality rather than a surgical failure of local tumor resection. Interestingly, many so called "recurrent" tumors are often found in locations fully remote from the original site of resection.

Partial Nephrectomy for Local Recurrence

Owing to the significant surgical challenges involved with reoperative renal surgery for recurrent disease, there are few publications available to guide patients and their urologists.[103–105] Johnson and colleagues[90] at NCI reviewed 51 planned repeat partial nephrectomies in 47 patients with local recurrence. A total of 40 perioperative complications occurred. Most of these complications did not result in long-term disability, but one subject suffered an intraoperative myocardial infarction and died postoperatively, and 3 subjects lost a renal unit. Despite the increased degree of perioperative morbidity associated with repeat NSS, only 3 patients (5.8%) in Johnson and colleagues'[90] series required renal replacement therapy; a number that would have been markedly higher if radical nephrectomy had been performed, as one-third of the surgeries in their cohort were performed on a solitary kidney (**Table 1**).

Table 1
Comparison of perioperative outcomes by partial nephrectomy type

Type of Partial Nephrectomy	Johnson et al,[90] 2008 Repeat	Bratslavsky et al,[89] 2008 Salvage	Kowalczyk et al,[111] 2009 Post-RFA	Fadahunsi et al,[75] 2011 ≥20 Tumors
Number of patients	47	11	13	30
Number of partial nephrectomies	51	13	16	34
Median tumors removed (range)	7 (1–55)	5 (1–27)	7 (2–40)	26.5 (20–70)
Median EBL, mL (range)	1800 (50–21,500)	2100 (200–12,000)	1500 (500–3500)	3500 (800–19,500)
Transfusion requirement (%)	38 (75)	10 (77)	8 (50)	30 (88.2)
Median units transfused (range)	2 (0–31)	4.5 (0–18)	4 (1–8)	6.5 (0–32)
Intraoperative complications:				
Visceral or vascular injury (%)	2 (4)	6 (46)	0	1 (3)
Ureteral injury (%)	1	0	1 (6)	0
Pleural injury (%)	NA	NA	5 (31)	16 (47)
Postoperative complications:				
Prolonged urine leak (%)	8 (15)	2 (15)	3 (19)	11 (32)
Permanent hemodialysis (%)	3 (6)	2 (15)	0	0
Renal unit loss (%)	3 (6)	3 (23)	0	1 (3)
Rhabdomyolysis (%)	0	1 (8)	1 (6)	2 (6)
Reoperation (%)	2 (4)	4 (36)	2 (13)	2 (6)
Cardiovascular events (%)	1 (2)	0	2 (13)	3 (9)

Abbreviations: EBL, estimated blood loss; NA, not available; RFA, radiofrequency ablation.

Bratslavsky and colleagues[89] studied a small cohort of patients who underwent 3 or more operations on the same renal unit, which they termed "salvage" partial nephrectomy. Major perioperative complications occurred in nearly half of patients; however, more than three-fourths of the renal units were saved with minimal changes in postoperative serum creatinine, creatinine clearance, and differential renal function. Salvage partial nephrectomy should therefore be considered a viable option for select patients with recurrent, multifocal, localized kidney cancer (see **Table 1**).

In many cases, the ablation may still be a viable option to treat the "recurrence"; however, the role of ablation for recurrent RCC may be limited, as the "recurrences" are usually multifocal and arise in different areas of the kidney. Although ablation may be successful for some of the newly formed "recurrent" tumors, other tumors may not be amenable to ablation because of tumor location next to the hilum or the ureter, or proximity to the adjacent organs. Therefore, the most optimal management of the multifocal tumors after previous partial nephrectomy has been a "maximal cleanout" to reset the next intervention as far back as possible by removing all visible tumors. Occasionally, if there is a solitary new tumor, or a very limited number of these recurrent tumors with all amenable to ablation, it may be reasonable to consider ablation as an alternative to repeat or salvage partial nephrectomy.

Partial Nephrectomy After Thermal Ablation

Thermal ablation, achieved via cryoablation (CA) or radiofrequency ablation (RFA), has been used to treat small renal masses since the late 1990s.[106] In patients with a sporadic T1a renal tumor, ablation is considered a recommendation in those with significant comorbidities.[2] In those with hereditary syndromes, ablation has been used in only a small number of patients. Series with a limited number of patients, have described ablation as the initial treatment, as well as in those with local recurrence.[107–110] For ablation failures, retreatment with another round of CA or RFA is an option; however, when a new lesion or a recurrence is not amenable to repeat ablation and extirpation is needed, partial nephrectomy can be extremely challenging.

Kowalczyk and colleagues[111] performed 16 partial nephrectomies on 13 patients after 18 prior RFA treatments (see **Table 1**). Three-quarters of cases were noted to have extensive scarring at the prior RFA site. Intraoperative complications included pleural injury and ureteral injury, whereas postoperative complications included urine leak and hemorrhage that required a return to the operating room for exploration and control. Rhabdomyolysis, atrial fibrillation, and deep venous thrombosis were each seen in one patient; however, despite these serious complications, no renal units were lost and no patient required renal replacement therapy (RRT).

Partial Nephrectomy for More Than 20 Tumors

Fadahunsi and colleagues[75] evaluated the feasibility and outcomes of partial nephrectomy used to resect at least 20 tumors from a single renal unit during one operation. They identified 30 patients treated at NCI between 1998 and 2008 who underwent 34 partial nephrectomies with a median of 26.5 tumors removed.

Perioperative complications occurred in more than half of cases, with urine leak seen in nearly one-third of patients. Fifty-nine percent of surgeries were performed without hilar clamping. Median estimated blood loss was 3500 mL and 88% of patients received intraoperative blood transfusions with an additional 12% receiving transfusions postoperatively. Although estimated glomerular function decreased 3 months postoperatively (67 vs 59 mL/min/1.73 m^2, $P<.001$), all patients were able to avoid RRT.

One patient (3%) developed metastatic disease 5 months after surgery, although 8 months before that diagnosis he had undergone a contralateral partial nephrectomy that removed 17 tumors, the largest of which measured 5.5 cm, making it difficult to determine the cause of the metastatic event. No deaths were reported in this cohort and only one renal unit was lost, indicating that this type of aggressive partial nephrectomy is technically feasible and provides adequate renal preservation and oncologic control at a median follow-up of 52 months. Functional and oncologic outcomes of NCI partial nephrectomies for multifocal and hereditary RCC are summarized in **Tables 2** and **3**, respectively.

Long-Term Outcomes

Singer and colleagues[112] recently described the renal functional and oncologic outcomes of patients with bilateral renal masses managed surgically at NCI who had at least 10 years of postoperative follow-up. They identified a cohort of 128 patients who had undergone bilateral renal surgery with a median of 3 operations per person.

Table 2
Renal functional outcomes

Procedure	First Author, Year	n	Units Lost (%)	Δ in Cr mg/dL	Δ in Cr Clearance mL/min	% Δ in Cr Clearance
Initial partial nephrectomy	Herring et al,[113] 2001	65	5%	0.01	NA	NA
Post RFA partial	Kowalczyk et al,[111] 2009	16	0%	0.1	−10	−11%
Partial for >20 tumors	Fadahunsi et al,[75] 2011	34	3%	0.2	−7	−11%
Repeat partial nephrectomy	Johnson et al,[90] 2008	51	6%	0.19	−10	−11%
Repeat partial on a solitary unit	Liu et al,[114] 2010	24	13%	0.2	−8	−15%
Salvage partial nephrectomy	Bratslavsky et al,[89] 2008	13	23%	0.2	−16	−17%

Abbreviations: Cr, creatine; NA, not available; RFA, radiofrequency ablation.

Table 3
Renal cell carcinoma oncologic outcomes

Procedure	First Author, Year	Median Follow-up, mo	Metastasis-Free Survival, %	Overall Survival, %
Initial partial nephrectomy	Herring et al,[113] 2001	30	100	100
Partial for >20 tumors	Fadahunsi et al,[75] 2011	50	92	92
Repeat partial nephrectomy	Johnson et al,[90] 2008	56	94	98
Repeat partial on a solitary unit	Liu et al,[114] 2010	69	95	90
Salvage partial nephrectomy	Bratslavsky et al,[89] 2008	25	100	100

Sixty-eight percent of the cohort had repeat surgery on the same renal unit, with a median time between interventions of 6.2 years. At a median follow-up of 16 years, overall survival was 88%, RCC-specific survival was 97%, and metastasis-free survival was 88%. The most recent calculated median estimated glomerular filtration rate was 57 mL/min/1.73 m^2 for the entire cohort. More than 95% of patients avoided RRT. This work has demonstrated that at a minimum of 10 years after initial surgery, and despite the need for repeat surgical interventions on the same kidney, NSS allows for excellent oncologic and functional outcomes in selected patients.

SUMMARY

Although the management of sporadic renal tumors is challenging enough, dealing with those with bilateral, multifocal, and hereditary kidney cancer adds an additional level of complexity. A clinician managing this patient population must understand the hereditary syndromes and the genetic testing available. If affected with a germline mutation, other family members should be offered screening and surveillance if they are found to be carriers of a germline mutation. In patients without an identifiable genetic syndrome but with bilateral, multifocal renal tumors, similar management to those with hereditary syndromes is used. The goal of management in these patients is to prevent RCC dissemination, maximize renal functional outcomes, and minimize morbidity to the patient. To accomplish these goals, treating physicians must be familiar with enucleative surgery, complex or multiple tumor partial nephrectomy, complex renal reconstruction, reoperative renal surgery, and active surveillance strategies. With proper management, most patients affected with bilateral, multifocal, or hereditary RCC can have a long life expectancy while maintaining adequate renal function.

REFERENCES

1. Cooperberg MR, Mallin K, Kane CJ, et al. Treatment trends for stage I renal cell carcinoma. J Urol 2011;186(2):394–9.
2. Campbell SC, Novick AC, Belldegrun A, et al. Guideline for management of the clinical T1 renal mass. J Urol 2009;182(4):1271–9.
3. Bratslavsky G, Linehan WM. Long-term management of bilateral, multifocal, recurrent renal carcinoma. Nat Rev Urol 2010;7(5):267–75.
4. Klatte T, Wunderlich H, Patard JJ, et al. Clinicopathological features and prognosis of synchronous bilateral renal cell carcinoma: an international multicentre experience. BJU Int 2007;100(1):21–5.
5. Wunderlich H, Schlichter A, Zermann D, et al. Multifocality in renal cell carcinoma: a bilateral event? Urol Int 1999;63(3):160–3.
6. Blute ML, Itano NB, Cheville JC, et al. The effect of bilaterality, pathological features and surgical outcome in nonhereditary renal cell carcinoma. J Urol 2003;169(4):1276–81.
7. Klatte T, Patard JJ, Wunderlich H, et al. Metachronous bilateral renal cell carcinoma: risk assessment, prognosis and relevance of the primary-free interval. J Urol 2007;177(6):2081–6 [discussion: 2086–7].
8. Rabbani F, Herr HW, Almahmeed T, et al. Temporal change in risk of metachronous contralateral renal cell carcinoma: influence of tumor characteristics and demographic factors. J Clin Oncol 2002; 20(9):2370–5.
9. Lau WK, Blute ML, Weaver AL, et al. Matched comparison of radical nephrectomy vs nephron-sparing surgery in patients with unilateral renal cell carcinoma and a normal contralateral kidney. Mayo Clin Proc 2000;75(12):1236–42.
10. Whang M, O'Toole K, Bixon R, et al. The incidence of multifocal renal cell carcinoma in patients who are candidates for partial nephrectomy. J Urol 1995;154(3):968–70 [discussion: 970–1].

11. Schlichter A, Schubert R, Werner W, et al. How accurate is diagnostic imaging in determination of size and multifocality of renal cell carcinoma as a prerequisite for nephron-sparing surgery? Urol Int 2000;64(4):192–7.

12. Nissenkorn I, Bernheim J. Multicentricity in renal cell carcinoma. J Urol 1995;153(3 Pt 1):620–2.

13. Minervini A, Serni S, Giubilei G, et al. Multiple ipsilateral renal tumors: retrospective analysis of surgical and oncological results of tumor enucleation vs radical nephrectomy. Eur J Surg Oncol 2009;35(5):521–6.

14. Rabbani F, McLoughlin MG. Parameters predictive of multicentricity in renal cell carcinoma. Can J Urol 1997;4(3):406–11.

15. Cheng WS, Farrow GM, Zincke H. The incidence of multicentricity in renal cell carcinoma. J Urol 1991; 146(5):1221–3.

16. Mukamel E, Konichezky M, Engelstein D, et al. Incidental small renal tumors accompanying clinically overt renal cell carcinoma. J Urol 1988;140(1): 22–4.

17. Kletscher BA, Qian J, Bostwick DG, et al. Prospective analysis of multifocality in renal cell carcinoma: influence of histological pattern, grade, number, size, volume and deoxyribonucleic acid ploidy. J Urol 1995;153(3 Pt 2):904–6.

18. Gudbjartsson T, Jonasdottir TJ, Thoroddsen A, et al. A population-based familial aggregation analysis indicates genetic contribution in a majority of renal cell carcinomas. Int J Cancer 2002;100(4):476–9.

19. Purdue MP, Johansson M, Zelenika D, et al. Genome-wide association study of renal cell carcinoma identifies two susceptibility loci on 2p21 and 11q13.3. Nat Genet 2011;43(1):60–5.

20. Wu X, Scelo G, Purdue MP, et al. A genome-wide association study identifies a novel susceptibility locus for renal cell carcinoma on 12p11.23. Hum Mol Genet 2012;21(2):456–62.

21. Hosoe S, Brauch H, Latif F, et al. Localization of the von Hippel-Lindau disease gene to a small region of chromosome 3. Genomics 1990;8(4):634–40.

22. Latif F, Tory K, Gnarra J, et al. Identification of the von Hippel-Lindau disease tumor suppressor gene. Science 1993;260(5112):1317–20.

23. Gnarra JR, Tory K, Weng Y, et al. Mutations of the VHL tumour suppressor gene in renal carcinoma. Nat Genet 1994;7(1):85–90.

24. Lonser RR, Glenn GM, Walther M, et al. von Hippel-Lindau disease. Lancet 2003;361(9374):2059–67.

25. Choyke PL, Filling-Katz MR, Shawker TH, et al. von Hippel-Lindau disease: radiologic screening for visceral manifestations. Radiology 1990;174(3 Pt 1): 815–20.

26. Birt AR, Hogg GR, Dube WJ. Hereditary multiple fibrofolliculomas with trichodiscomas and acrochordons. Arch Dermatol 1977;113(12):1674–7.

27. Roth JS, Rabinowitz AD, Benson M, et al. Bilateral renal cell carcinoma in the Birt-Hogg-Dube syndrome. J Am Acad Dermatol 1993;29(6):1055–6.

28. Toro JR, Glenn G, Duray P, et al. Birt-Hogg-Dube syndrome: a novel marker of kidney neoplasia. Arch Dermatol 1999;135(10):1195–202.

29. Schmidt LS, Warren MB, Nickerson ML, et al. Birt-Hogg-Dube syndrome, a genodermatosis associated with spontaneous pneumothorax and kidney neoplasia, maps to chromosome 17p11.2. Am J Hum Genet 2001;69(4):876–82.

30. Nickerson ML, Warren MB, Toro JR, et al. Mutations in a novel gene lead to kidney tumors, lung wall defects, and benign tumors of the hair follicle in patients with the Birt-Hogg-Dube syndrome. Cancer Cell 2002;2(2):157–64.

31. Schmidt LS, Nickerson ML, Warren MB, et al. Germline BHD-mutation spectrum and phenotype analysis of a large cohort of families with Birt-Hogg-Dube syndrome. Am J Hum Genet 2005; 76(6):1023–33.

32. Pavlovich CP, Walther MM, Eyler RA, et al. Renal tumors in the Birt-Hogg-Dube syndrome. Am J Surg Pathol 2002;26(12):1542–52.

33. Pavlovich CP, Grubb RL 3rd, Hurley K, et al. Evaluation and management of renal tumors in the Birt-Hogg-Dube syndrome. J Urol 2005;173(5):1482–6.

34. Kloepfer HW, Krafchuk J, Derbes V, et al. Hereditary multiple leiomyoma of the skin. Am J Hum Genet 1958;10(1):48–52.

35. Reed WB, Walker R, Horowitz R. Cutaneous leiomyomata with uterine leiomyomata. Acta Derm Venereol 1973;53(5):409–16.

36. Launonen V, Vierimaa O, Kiuru M, et al. Inherited susceptibility to uterine leiomyomas and renal cell cancer. Proc Natl Acad Sci U S A 2001;98(6):3387–92.

37. Merino MJ, Torres-Cabala C, Pinto P, et al. The morphologic spectrum of kidney tumors in hereditary leiomyomatosis and renal cell carcinoma (HLRCC) syndrome. Am J Surg Pathol 2007; 31(10):1578–85.

38. Alam NA, Bevan S, Churchman M, et al. Localization of a gene (MCUL1) for multiple cutaneous leiomyomata and uterine fibroids to chromosome 1q42.3-q43. Am J Hum Genet 2001;68(5):1264–9.

39. Tomlinson IP, Alam NA, Rowan AJ, et al. Germline mutations in FH predispose to dominantly inherited uterine fibroids, skin leiomyomata and papillary renal cell cancer. Nat Genet 2002;30(4):406–10.

40. Kiuru M, Launonen V, Hietala M, et al. Familial cutaneous leiomyomatosis is a two-hit condition associated with renal cell cancer of characteristic histopathology. Am J Pathol 2001;159(3):825–9.

41. Vanharanta S, Pollard PJ, Lehtonen HJ, et al. Distinct expression profile in fumarate-hydratase-deficient uterine fibroids. Hum Mol Genet 2006; 15(1):97–103.

42. Grubb RL 3rd, Franks ME, Toro J, et al. Hereditary leiomyomatosis and renal cell cancer: a syndrome associated with an aggressive form of inherited renal cancer. J Urol 2007;177(6):2074–9 [discussion: 2079–80].

43. Zbar B, Tory K, Merino M, et al. Hereditary papillary renal cell carcinoma. J Urol 1994;151(3):561–6.

44. Schmidt L, Duh FM, Chen F, et al. Germline and somatic mutations in the tyrosine kinase domain of the MET proto-oncogene in papillary renal carcinomas. Nat Genet 1997;16(1):68–73.

45. Zhuang Z, Park WS, Pack S, et al. Trisomy 7-harbouring non-random duplication of the mutant MET allele in hereditary papillary renal carcinomas. Nat Genet 1998;20(1):66–9.

46. Choueri TK, Vaishampayan UN, Rosenberg JE, et al. A Phase II and biomarker study (MET111644) of the dual MET/VEGFR-2 inhibitor foretinib in patients with sporadic and hereditary papillary renal cell carcinoma: final efficacy, safety, and PD results. 2012, ASCO GU Cancer Symposium. San Francisco (CA) [abstract 355].

47. Astuti D, Latif F, Dallol A, et al. Gene mutations in the succinate dehydrogenase subunit SDHB cause susceptibility to familial pheochromocytoma and to familial paraganglioma. Am J Hum Genet 2001; 69(1):49–54.

48. Neumann HP, Pawlu C, Peczkowska M, et al. Distinct clinical features of paraganglioma syndromes associated with SDHB and SDHD gene mutations. JAMA 2004;292(8):943–51.

49. Ricketts C, Woodward ER, Killick P, et al. Germline SDHB mutations and familial renal cell carcinoma. J Natl Cancer Inst 2008;100(17):1260–2.

50. Gill AJ, Pachter NS, Chou A, et al. Renal tumors associated with germline SDHB mutation show distinctive morphology. Am J Surg Pathol 2011; 35(10):1578–85.

51. European Chromosome 16 Tuberous Sclerosis Consortium. Identification and characterization of the tuberous sclerosis gene on chromosome 16. Cell 1993;75(7):1305–15.

52. van Slegtenhorst M, de Hoogt R, Hermans C, et al. Identification of the tuberous sclerosis gene TSC1 on chromosome 9q34. Science 1997;277(5327):805–8.

53. Clarke A, Hancock E, Kingswood C, et al. End-stage renal failure in adults with the tuberous sclerosis complex. Nephrol Dial Transplant 1999;14(4): 988–91.

54. Bjornsson J, Short MP, Kwiatkowski DJ, et al. Tuberous sclerosis-associated renal cell carcinoma. Clinical, pathological, and genetic features. Am J Pathol 1996;149(4):1201–8.

55. Duffy K, Al-Saleem T, Karbowniczek M, et al. Mutational analysis of the von Hippel Lindau gene in clear cell renal carcinomas from tuberous sclerosis complex patients. Mod Pathol 2002;15(3):205–10.

56. Dechet CB, Bostwick DG, Blute ML, et al. Renal oncocytoma: multifocality, bilateralism, metachronous tumor development and coexistent renal cell carcinoma. J Urol 1999;162(1):40–2.

57. Perez-Ordonez B, Hamed G, Campbell S, et al. Renal oncocytoma: a clinicopathologic study of 70 cases. Am J Surg Pathol 1997;21(8):871–83.

58. Boris RS, Benhammou J, Merino M, et al. The impact of germline BHD mutation on histological concordance and clinical treatment of patients with bilateral renal masses and known unilateral oncocytoma. J Urol 2011;185(6):2050–5.

59. Patel AR, Lee BH, Campbell SC, et al. Bilateral synchronous sporadic renal tumors: pathologic concordance and clinical implications. Urology 2011;78(5):1095–9.

60. Tickoo SK, Reuter VE, Amin MB, et al. Renal oncocytosis: a morphologic study of fourteen cases. Am J Surg Pathol 1999;23(9):1094–101.

61. Farkas LM, Szekely JG, Karatson A. Bilateral, multifocal renal oncocytomatosis with rapid progression leading to renal insufficiency. Nephrol Dial Transplant 1999;14(9):2262–3.

62. Adamy A, Lowrance WT, Yee DS, et al. Renal oncocytosis: management and clinical outcomes. J Urol 2011;185(3):795–801.

63. Weirich G, Glenn G, Junker K, et al. Familial renal oncocytoma: clinicopathological study of 5 families. J Urol 1998;160(2):335–40.

64. Black J, Rotellar C, Rakowski TA, et al. Bilateral nephrectomy and dialysis as an option for patients with bilateral renal cancer. Nephron 1988;49(2): 150–3.

65. Calne RY. Treatment of bilateral hypernephromas by nephrectomy, excision of tumour, and autotransplantation. Report of three cases. Lancet 1973; 2(7839):1164–7.

66. Clark JE. Transplantation for bilateral renal tumors. JAMA 1970;211(8):1379.

67. Jochimsen PR, Braunstein PM, Najarian JS. Renal allotransplantation for bilateral renal tumors. JAMA 1969;210(9):1721–4.

68. Fetner CD, Barilla DE, Scott T, et al. Bilateral renal cell carcinoma in von Hippel-Lindau syndrome: treatment with staged bilateral nephrectomy and hemodialysis. J Urol 1977;117(4):534–6.

69. Mullin EM, White RD, Peterson LJ, et al. Bilateral renal carcinoma in von Hippel-Lindau disease. Urology 1976;8(5):475–8.

70. Goldfarb DA, Neumann HP, Penn I, et al. Results of renal transplantation in patients with renal cell carcinoma and von Hippel-Lindau disease. Transplantation 1997;64(12):1726–9.

71. U S Renal Data System (USRDS). USRDS 2010 Annual data report. Minneapolis (MN): USRDS; 2010.

72. Stiles KP, Moffatt MJ, Agodoa LY, et al. Renal cell carcinoma as a cause of end-stage renal disease

in the United States: patient characteristics and survival. Kidney Int 2003;64(1):247–53.

73. Ajithkumar TV, Parkinson CA, Butler A, et al. Management of solid tumours in organ-transplant recipients. Lancet Oncol 2007;8(10):921–32.

74. Kasiske BL, Cangro CB, Hariharan S, et al; American Society of Transplantation. The evaluation of renal transplant candidates: clinical practice guidelines. Am J Transplant 2001;(Suppl 2):1–95.

75. Fadahunsi AT, Sanford T, Linehan WM, et al. Feasibility and outcomes of partial nephrectomy for resection of at least 20 tumors in a single renal unit. J Urol 2011;185(1):49–53.

76. Russo P. Open partial nephrectomy: an essential operation with an expanding role. Curr Opin Urol 2007;17(5):309–15.

77. Singer EA, Bratslavsky G. Management of locally recurrent kidney cancer. Curr Urol Rep 2010; 11(1):15–21.

78. Duffey BG, Choyke PL, Glenn G, et al. The relationship between renal tumor size and metastases in patients with von Hippel-Lindau disease. J Urol 2004;172(1):63–5.

79. Walther MM, Choyke PL, Glenn G, et al. Renal cancer in families with hereditary renal cancer: prospective analysis of a tumor size threshold for renal parenchymal sparing surgery. J Urol 1999; 161(5):1475–9.

80. Sutherland SE, Resnick MI, Maclennan GT, et al. Does the size of the surgical margin in partial nephrectomy for renal cell cancer really matter? J Urol 2002;167(1):61–4.

81. Carini M, Minervini A, Masieri L, et al. Simple enucleation for the treatment of PT1a renal cell carcinoma: our 20-year experience. Eur Urol 2006;50(6):1263–8 [discussion: 1269–71].

82. Carini M, Minervini A, Lapini A, et al. Simple enucleation for the treatment of renal cell carcinoma between 4 and 7 cm in greatest dimension: progression and long-term survival. J Urol 2006; 175(6):2022–6 [discussion: 2026].

83. Minervini A, Ficarra V, Rocco F, et al. Simple enucleation is equivalent to traditional partial nephrectomy for renal cell carcinoma: results of a nonrandomized, retrospective, comparative study. J Urol 2011;185(5):1604–10.

84. Rini BI. Metastatic renal cell carcinoma: many treatment options, one patient. J Clin Oncol 2009; 27(19):3225–34.

85. Boris R, Proano M, Linehan WM, et al. Initial experience with robot assisted partial nephrectomy for multiple renal masses. J Urol 2009; 182(4):1280–6.

86. Flum AS, Wolf JS Jr. Laparoscopic partial nephrectomy for multiple ipsilateral renal tumors using a tailored surgical approach. J Endourol 2010; 24(4):557–61.

87. Steinberg AP, Kilciler M, Abreu SC, et al. Laparoscopic nephron-sparing surgery for two or more ipsilateral renal tumors. Urology 2004;64(2): 255–8.

88. Boris RS, Gupta G, Linehan WM, et al. Feasibility and outcomes of laparoscopic renal intervention after prior open ipsilateral retroperitoneal surgery. In: Society of Urologic Oncology, Winter Meeting. Besthesda (MD), 2010.

89. Bratslavsky G, Liu JJ, Johnson AD, et al. Salvage partial nephrectomy for hereditary renal cancer: feasibility and outcomes. J Urol 2008;179(1):67–70.

90. Johnson A, Sudarshan S, Liu J, et al. Feasibility and outcomes of repeat partial nephrectomy. J Urol 2008;180(1):89–93 [discussion: 93].

91. Sporer A, Seebode JJ. Study of renal blood supply and its implication in renal pelvic surgery. Urology 1981;17(1):18–21.

92. Walther MM, Choyke PL, Hayes W, et al. Evaluation of color Doppler intraoperative ultrasound in parenchymal sparing renal surgery. J Urol 1994; 152(6 Pt 1):1984–7.

93. Choyke PL, Daryanani K. Intraoperative ultrasound of the kidney. Ultrasound Q 2001;17(4):245–53.

94. Choyke PL, Pavlovich CP, Daryanani KD, et al. Intraoperative ultrasound during renal parenchymal sparing surgery for hereditary renal cancers: a 10-year experience. J Urol 2001;165(2):397–400.

95. Shuch B, Lam JS, Belldegrun AS. Open partial nephrectomy for the treatment of renal cell carcinoma. Curr Urol Rep 2006;7(1):31–8.

96. Thompson RH, Lane BR, Lohse CM, et al. Comparison of warm ischemia versus no ischemia during partial nephrectomy on a solitary kidney. Eur Urol 2010;58(3):331–6.

97. Thompson RH, Lane BR, Lohse CM, et al. Every minute counts when the renal hilum is clamped during partial nephrectomy. Eur Urol 2010;58(3):340–5.

98. Lane BR, Russo P, Uzzo RG, et al. Comparison of cold and warm ischemia during partial nephrectomy in 660 solitary kidneys reveals predominant role of nonmodifiable factors in determining ultimate renal function. J Urol 2011; 185(2):421–7.

99. Thompson RH, Frank I, Lohse CM, et al. The impact of ischemia time during open nephron sparing surgery on solitary kidneys: a multi-institutional study. J Urol 2007;177(2):471–6.

100. Walther MM, Thompson N, Linehan W. Enucleation procedures in patients with multiple hereditary renal tumors. World J Urol 1995;13(4):248–50.

101. Singer EA, Bratslavsky G, Middelton L, et al. Impact of genetics on the diagnosis and treatment of renal cancer. Curr Urol Rep 2011;12(1):47–55.

102. Tsivian M, Moreira DM, Caso JR, et al. Predicting occult multifocality of renal cell carcinoma. Eur Urol 2010;58(1):118–26.

103. Ansari MS, Gupta NP, Kumar P. von Hippel-Lindau disease with bilateral multiple renal cell carcinoma managed by right radical nephrectomy and left repeat partial nephrectomy. Int Urol Nephrol 2003;35(4):471–3.

104. Novick AC, Streem SB. Long-term follow-up after nephron sparing surgery for renal cell carcinoma in von Hippel-Lindau disease. J Urol 1992;147(6): 1488–90.

105. Steinbach F, Novick AC, Zincke H, et al. Treatment of renal cell carcinoma in von Hippel-Lindau disease: a multicenter study. J Urol 1995;153(6): 1812–6.

106. Kunkle DA, Uzzo RG. Cryoablation or radiofrequency ablation of the small renal mass: a meta-analysis. Cancer 2008;113(10):2671–80.

107. Park BK, Kim CK. Percutaneous radio frequency ablation of renal tumors in patients with von Hippel-Lindau disease: preliminary results. J Urol 2010;183(5):1703–7.

108. Park SY, Park BK, Kim CK, et al. Percutaneous radiofrequency ablation of renal cell carcinomas in patients with von Hippel-Lindau disease previously undergoing a radical nephrectomy or repeated nephron-sparing surgery. Acta Radiol 2011;52(6):680–5.

109. Shingleton WB, Sewell PE Jr. Percutaneous renal cryoablation of renal tumors in patients with von Hippel-Lindau disease. J Urol 2002;167(3): 1268–70.

110. Yang B, Autorino R, Remer EM, et al. Probe ablation as salvage therapy for renal tumors in von Hippel-Lindau patients: the Cleveland Clinic experience with 3 years follow-up. Urol Oncol 2011. [Epub ahead of print].

111. Kowalczyk KJ, Hooper HB, Linehan WM, et al. Partial nephrectomy after previous radio frequency ablation: the National Cancer Institute experience. J Urol 2009;182(5):2158–63.

112. Singer EA, Vourganti S, Lin K, et al. Outcomes of patients with surgically treated bilateral renal masses and a minimum of 10 years of follow-up: the NCI experience. J Urol 2011;185(Suppl 4): e746.

113. Herring JC, Enquist EG, Chernoff A, et al. Parenchymal sparing surgery in patients with hereditary renal cell carcinoma: 10-year experience. J Urol 2001;165(3):777–81.

114. Liu NW, Khurana K, Sudarshan S, et al. Repeat partial nephrectomy on the solitary kidney: surgical, functional and oncological outcomes. J Urol 2010;183(5):1719–24.

Current Practice Patterns in the Surgical Management of Renal Cancer in the United States

Ganesh Sivarajan, MD[a], William Huang, MD[b],*

KEYWORDS

- Surgical management • Renal cancer • United States
- Current practice

INTRODUCTION AND EPIDEMIOLOGY

Renal cell carcinoma (RCC) accounts for approximately 3.5% of all malignancies and is the third most common cancer of the urinary tract.[1] In 2010 there were an estimated 58,240 incident cases and 8210 cancer-related deaths. RCC ranks seventh among the leading causes of cancer in men and ninth among the leading causes of cancer among women in the United States.[2] These figures also show an increasing incidence of RCC over the past few decades. Hollingsworth and colleagues[3] estimated that the age-adjusted incidence increased from 7.1 to 10.8 cases per 100,000 of US population between 1983 and 2002.

Both this increasing incidence as well as a concomitant downward migration in clinical stage and primary tumor size at presentation are at least partly attributable to the increasing use of cross-sectional abdominal imaging in the diagnosis of renal masses. It has been estimated that at least 48% to 66% of RCC diagnoses occur as a result of cross-sectional imaging in an otherwise asymptomatic patient.[4] Furthermore, the number of renal masses, both benign and malignant, discovered only at autopsy is declining, possibly because of increased detection before death.[5]

This increasing incidence of RCC and the parallel increase in the national nephrectomy rate over the last 2 decades are emblematic of the changing clinical presentation and behavior of these tumors.[3,6] Tumors are now heterogeneous in nature; 20% are entirely benign, with an additional 20% to 25% representing a potentially aggressive malignancy at the time of diagnosis.[7–10] The changing landscape in tumor diagnosis and tumor biology has also resulted in changes in the management of these renal masses.

OVERVIEW OF TREATMENT OPTIONS
Open Radical Nephrectomy

Robson[11] is generally credited with establishing open radical nephrectomy (ORN) as the gold standard intervention for management of organ-confined and locally advanced renal cortical tumors. Key components of this technique included removal of the entire kidney with all surrounding perinephric tissue, resection of the ipsilateral adrenal gland, and regional lymph node dissection. Although this operation remained the standard of care for renal masses for more than 40 years, the increasing incidence of smaller and lower-stage tumors in the modern day has led to an evolution in the surgical management of this disease; namely, an increased acceptance of nephron-sparing as well as minimally invasive approaches. However, ORN remains indicated

[a] Department of Urology, NYU Langone Medical Center, 2nd Floor, 150 East 32nd Street, New York, NY 10016, USA
[b] Department of Urology, NYU Langone Medical Center, NYU Cancer Institute, 150 East 32nd Street, New York, NY 10016, USA
* Corresponding author.
E-mail address: William.huang@nyumc.org

Urol Clin N Am 39 (2012) 149–160
doi:10.1016/j.ucl.2012.01.001

when nephron-sparing partial nephrectomy (PN) cannot be curative, such as instances of tumor thrombus, local invasion of surrounding organs, or significant lymphadenopathy.

Laparoscopic Radical Nephrectomy

Minimally invasive radical nephrectomy (RN) was first described by Clayman and colleagues[12] in the early 1990s. Although its increased technical demands compared with ORN initially limited its acceptance, improved convalescence with demonstrably similar cancer control outcomes have led to its acceptance as an alternative standard of care in patients who require RN for RCC.[13–16] Specifically, laparoscopic RN (LRN) has been linked to improved perioperative outcomes, including decreased blood loss, less pain, shorter length of stay, improved cosmesis, and faster return to work and normal activities.[16–18] Although LRN is considered the preferred approach only in patients with tumors that are not amenable to PN, the adoption of laparoscopy to RN has nevertheless been slow compared with other laparoscopic treatments.

PN

Nephron-sparing approaches, particularly PN, have become increasingly popular over the last decade. Historically, open PN has been the primary approach for nephron-sparing surgery (NSS), the benefits of which derive from the preservation of renal parenchyma and renal function. Although originally reserved for patients with absolute indications such as instances of bilateral RCC, RCC in a solitary kidney, or RCC in the setting of preexisting kidney disease,[19] it is now being routinely applied at tertiary-care centers for the management of localized renal tumors. This emphasis on tumor resection without compromising normal parenchyma is not without risk. PN, whether performed in open or laparoscopic fashion, is generally considered to be a more technically demanding operation than ORN or even LRN, with a resultant higher rate of complications such as hemorrhage, urinary fistula formation, ureteral obstruction, acute renal insufficiency, and infection.[20] However, technical considerations aside, it has been shown that PN reduces the risk of chronic kidney disease (CKD) compared with RN[21] and still achieves equivalent oncologic outcomes in tumors that measure less than 4 cm and even select tumors up to 7 cm in size.[22–25] Similar to RN, laparoscopic and now robotic approaches have been applied to PN over time.

Ablative Approaches

The technical challenges associated with the use of nephron-sparing approaches (eg, its learning curve, necessary emphasis on limiting ischemia time, and a reportedly higher morbidity/complication rate) have led to the proposal of needle-based ablative technology as an alternative treatment of small renal masses.[26] The efficacy of these ablative approaches is based on the placement of a needle or probe that, once placed into a target tumor, is able to induce a temperature-based lethality to all tissue within a fixed radius of ablation. This increasingly popular approach to the management of renal masses offers several advantages relative to surgery, including lower complication rates, shorter convalescence, absence of an ischemic insult, and the potential for outpatient management.[27,28] However, these advantages aside, at present the oncologic efficacy of ablative techniques remains largely unproved. Moreover, it has been suggested that these techniques should be restricted to smaller renal masses (eg, <3 cm), because larger tumors require multiple probes and carry a higher risk of incomplete ablation.[1] Another relative disadvantage to these techniques is the inability to acquire adequate tissue to provide complete pathologic staging of tumors or to confidently determine prognosis. Furthermore, an overall paucity of long-term oncologic data represents another notable drawback to this approach.

Active Surveillance

Although the perioperative morbidity associated with surgical intervention on renal masses has generally decreased as surgical techniques improve, some patients continue to be poor operative candidates or unwilling to accept the risks of surgical therapy. The mean age of patients undergoing RN and PN between 1988 and 2002 was 60.1 and 63.0 years, respectively.[4] Thus, as patients age, competing health risks begin to compromise overall survival more significantly than many incidentally found renal lesions.[29] A recent meta-analysis of 10 reports from the world literature evaluating untreated solid localized renal lesions reported a mean growth rate of 2.8 mm yearly and progression to metastatic disease in only 1% of cases at a mean follow-up of 38 months.[29] However, because there are still no large-scale, prospective data regarding the risks associated with observing small renal lesions, pursuing active surveillance of a renal lesion continues to represent a calculated risk by the treating physician and the affected patient.

TRENDS IN THE ADOPTION OF LRN VERSUS ORN

Although PN is now considered to be the reference standard for the management of small renal masses, RN remains indicated in instances in which PN is technically unfeasible. As outlined earlier, LRN has numerous demonstrable short-term benefits over ORN in perioperative outcomes such as decreased blood loss, shorter length of stay, less postoperative analgesia requirement, and faster return to work and normal activities.[16,17] Consideration of these advantages coupled with excellent long-term oncologic outcomes has established LRN as a clearly superior alternative to ORN for tumors that are not amenable to PN.[18,30–34] However, the adoption of this minimally invasive technique has been slow and incomplete since its initial introduction. Numerous population-based cohort studies have been done to assess any potential trends associated with the adoption of this technique throughout the United States.

The proportion of patients undergoing LRN has been generally increasing. Based on data abstracted from the Healthcare Cost and Use Project Nationwide Inpatient Sample (NIS) from 1991 to 2003, Miller and colleagues[35] found year of treatment to be the most robust determinant of laparoscopic use. Specifically, it was reported that patients treated between 2000 and 2003 were 11 times more likely to have undergone laparoscopic surgery than those treated from 1991 to 1993. Using a more contemporary series based on data abstracted from the Surveillance Epidemiology and End Results (SEER) program Medicare database between 1995 and 2005, Filson and colleagues[36] reported that this proportion increased from 1.4% in 1995 to 44.9% in 2005. Furthermore, analysis of the data with emphasis on trends in adoption by surgeons of LRN over time showed that the proportion of surgeons who performed at least 1 LRN in a given year increased from 1.7% in 1995 to 7.6% in 2000. After 2000, the rate of adoption accelerated considerably, reaching a peak of 42.6% in 2005. Despite these promising temporal trends, the adoption of laparoscopy for RCC has occurred at a slower rate than observed for other laparoscopic procedures such as cholecystectomy and fundoplication, both of which had surpassed open surgery (>50% of cases) within 5 years of their introduction.[37,38]

Factors Influencing the Adoption of RN

Tumor characteristics

These population-based cohort studies have also identified trends in the use of laparoscopy based on differences in tumor characteristics. For example, receipt of LRN has been shown to be twice as likely for tumors less than 4 cm in size than for those greater than 7 cm (24% vs 12%).[36] This finding is particularly puzzling

considering that the results of a survey-based study suggested that 57% of urologists would offer laparoscopic surgery to a hypothetical patient presenting with a 6-cm organ-confined renal mass.[39] Disparities in the use of laparoscopy have also been noted from tumor histology; however, these findings are of unclear significance because histology is frequently unknown at the time of surgical intervention.[36]

Patient demographics

Several disparities in the use of laparoscopy have also been noted based on differences in patient characteristics. In their analysis of SEER data abstracted from 1995 to 2005, Filson and colleagues[36] noted that whites were statistically significantly more likely to receive LRN than Hispanics (20% vs 12%). Furthermore, the investigators noted that those of high socioeconomic status were more likely to receive LRN than those of low socioeconomic status. In a similar vein, analysis of NIS data showed that those with private/health maintenance organization (HMO) insurance were more likely to undergo laparoscopic intervention compared with those with Medicare. In addition, those undergoing elective nephrectomy were more likely to receive laparoscopy than those undergoing urgent/emergent intervention.[35]

Hospital-related and surgeon-related factors

The application of laparoscopy seems to differ in a variety of hospital-based factors as well. More specifically, a greater propensity toward laparoscopy occurs in urban compared with rural hospitals as well as in teaching compared with nonteaching hospitals.[35] In addition, laparoscopy seems to be more commonly used in hospitals with a not-for-profit financial status compared with those that are for-profit.[35] However, perhaps most telling of all is the association between the nephrectomy volume of a hospital and the frequency of laparoscopic nephrectomy. Miller and colleagues reported that the greatest proportion of laparoscopic use was observed in patients treated at teaching hospitals with an overall high annual nephrectomy volume and in patients treated between 2000 and 2003. Consequently, the investigators postulated that the acceleration in the adoption of laparoscopy occurring after the year 2000 was the primary result of the expanded use of oncologic renal laparoscopy in a select group of medical centers (ie, high-volume, urban, teaching hospitals) and did not therefore indicate widespread diffusion of laparoscopic management of renal tumors throughout the United States.[35]

A host of surgeon-related factors seem to play a role in determining whether or not laparoscopy is used for renal masses. In 2008, using SEER data abstracted from 1997 to 2002, Miller and colleagues[40] concluded that the percentage of variance among the use of laparoscopy attributable to unmeasured surgeon factors was substantially greater than that attributable to tumor size or patient demographics. Attempts to characterize these surgeon factors have elucidated that LRN is more likely among urologists who work in larger organizations (medical schools or HMOs), those who practice in urban environments, and those with a major academic affiliation.[36]

Although the underuse of laparoscopy for management of renal tumors has been a matter of great concern over the last decade, the barriers to its widespread use remain unknown. The slow rate of adoption over the last 20 years is particularly perplexing when it is considered that within 3 years of the introduction of laparoscopic cholecystectomy, it was being used in more than 50% of cases nationwide and in up to 70% of cases by 4 years.[38] Several potential reasons for this conspicuously slow rate of dissemination have been suggested, such as differences in market forces, motivations of physicians to provide innovative therapies, patient preferences, the steepness of the learning curve, or the competing desire to offer NSS; however, more research on this matter is required to draw concrete conclusions.

TRENDS IN THE ADOPTION OF PN

In 2009, the American Urological Association issued guidelines from panel consensus establishing surgical excision by PN as a reference standard for the management of clinical T1 RCC.[41] These guidelines were based on several reports heralding equivalent long-term cancer-specific survival outcomes for PN and RN among clinical stage T1a and T1b renal tumors.[24,42–44] The primary benefit of PN over RN is rooted in the preservation of normal renal parenchyma and thus renal function. RCC has been estimated to be responsible for 0.6% of cases of end-stage renal disease in the United States.[45] Furthermore, within the last decade, a higher incidence of CKD in patients treated with RN as opposed to PN has been reported.[46,47] It also seems likely, for these same reasons, that PN may also reduce the risk of adverse cardiovascular events and premature death compared with RN.[21,48,49]

Despite the benefits of PN and the evidently equivalent oncologic outcomes, it has been suggested that PN remains underused in the treatment of small renal masses in the United States. Although some tertiary medical centers have reported PN rates approaching 90% for T1a renal tumors,[50,51] population-based studies suggest a lower estimated overall rate of 20% to 40% of all nephrectomies.[52,53]

There is a strong case for a persistent underuse of PN. Evidence of an underuse of PN nationwide can be clearly seen in **Fig. 1**, which depicts both the national PN and RN rates for renal masses less than 4 cm in size abstracted from SEER data as well as the PN and RN rates at our own tertiary-care institution. The reasons for this apparent underuse have been a matter of great concern, and thus several population-based cohort studies have been conducted in an effort to identify which factors are associated with the use of PN versus RN in the United States.

Factors Influencing the Adoption of PN

The most robust factor associated with the rate of PN has been the passage of time, because multiple investigators have reported increasing annual rates of PN over the last 2 decades. For example, from SEER data abstracted from

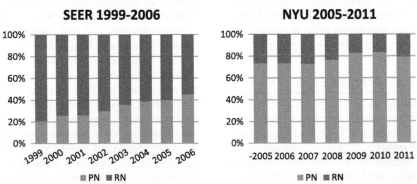

Fig. 1. Trends in use of RN versus PN. (*Data from* Dulabon LM, Lowrance WT, Russo P, et al. Trends in renal tumor surgery delivery within the United States. Cancer 2010;116(10):2316–21.)

between 1988 and 2001, Miller and colleagues[53] reported that the use of PN progressively increased for all tumors less than 7 cm in size. Specifically, a patient diagnosed in 2001 was nearly 5 times more likely to undergo PN than a patient diagnosed in 1988. More contemporary series have confirmed that this gradual increase in PN use for RCC has continued to the present day. Dulabon and colleagues,[52] using more recent SEER data, reported that the PN/RN ratio increased in statistically significant fashion between 1996 and 2006. Using NIS data from 2003 to 2008, Kim and colleagues[54] described a 90% increase in the annualized rate of PN per 100,000 individuals. However, despite these gradual increases, the investigators found that the overall rate of PN throughout the United States remained remarkably low. Even in 2008, PNs represented only 25.1% of all nephrectomy cases in the United States.[54] Furthermore, these small increases in PN use do not seem to be reflected uniformly across different patient populations, surgeon populations, and hospitals.

Tumor size

A disparity in the PN rate between tumors of varying size has been described in the literature. In general, from SEER data from 1999 to 2006, it has been reported that for each 1-cm increase in tumor size, there was an associated 47% lower odds of undergoing PN.[52] Similarly, the adoption of PN has therefore occurred most swiftly among patients with the smallest of tumors. In 1988 to 1989, 14% of tumors less than 2 cm underwent PN versus RN. This proportion had increased to 42% by 2000 to 2001.[53] More recent data even suggest that between 2002 and 2004, the rate of PN exceeded that of RN in renal masses less than 2 cm.[55]

By contrast, a slower rate of adoption has occurred for larger tumors. Among patients with tumors less than 4 cm in greatest dimension, only 5% underwent PN between 1988 and 1989; this had increased to only 20% by 2001 to 2002. Furthermore, over the same period, these T1a tumors were 3.8 times more likely to be treated with PN than T1b tumors.[53] The PN rate finally exceeded 50% in 2004 in these T1a tumors.[55]

Although the increasing rates of PN for very small renal tumors are promising, they still represent a gross underuse of the procedure, because PN is generally believed to offer equivalent oncologic outcomes in all tumors that measure less than 4 cm and even in select tumors up to 7 cm in size.[22–25] When T1b tumors are considered, both the PN rate and the rate of adoption over time are even lower. Using SEER data,

Baillargeon-Gagne and colleagues[55] showed that the PN rate for T1b tumors increased from 2.0% in 1989 to 10.0% in 2004. However, the proportion of overall patients with RCC undergoing PN between 2000 and 2002 was only 12.3%.

Nephrometry score

Although tumor size has certainly been reported to affect the likelihood of receiving PN, it is not the only tumor characteristic that has preoperative value in the assessment of renal masses. A nephrometry scoring system can be used to grade the complexity of a tumor by its size, exophytic versus endophytic nature, and anatomic position. Although it has been reported that a low complexity nephrometry score increases the likelihood of PN in some single-institution series,[56,57] this finding has never been assessed for validation in a large population-based cohort study. The impact and usefulness of the preoperative nephrometry score in guiding the surgical management of renal tumors remains an interesting question, which has yet to be definitively answered.

Age

There have been multiple reports of disparities among PN rates based on patient age. For example, NIS data abstracted from 1988 to 2002 suggested that patients older than 72 years were statistically significantly less likely to undergo PN compared with those 72 years or younger.[4] Even when considering only NIS data from 1998 to 2002, Porter and Lin[58] found that the odds of undergoing PN, compared with RN, decreased with each advancing age group from age less than 40 years, to age 40 to 59 years, to age 60 to 79 years, and those 80 years and older. More contemporary NIS data abstracted from 2003 to 2008 confirmed that patients aged 70 years or older were, in multivariate analysis, still approximately half as likely (odds ratio [OR] 0.51, $P<.001$) to undergo PN compared with their younger counterparts.[54] Analysis of SEER data from between 1998 and 2001 also indicated that patients treated with PN were significantly younger than those treated with RN (mean age 60.3 vs 62.5, $P<.01$).[53] This disparity was confirmed in more contemporary SEER data indicating that even between 1999 and 2006, those older than 70 years were significantly less likely to undergo PN compared with their younger counterparts.[52] A significantly higher rate of PN among younger patients compared with older counterparts has been reported in European populations as well.[51,59]

This age-based bias toward RN has been postulated by some to be the result of physician preference because it is thought to have fewer perioperative complications than PN. The disparity may be further perpetuated by the belief that the potential benefits of PN do not necessarily extend to the elderly population.[52,60,61] However, the validity of this logic has been called into question by data suggesting that both RN and a sudden decrease in glomerular filtration rate (GFR) are independent predictors of premature death in elderly patients.[49,62] Furthermore, PN reduces the risk of overtreating benign and indolent renal tumors in the elderly population who have lower GFR rates at baseline. However, theories that attempt to explain the bias against elderly patients in the use of PN are speculative, because no firm evidence to explain the disparity exists.

Gender

Differences in PN use between patients of opposite genders has become a matter of increasing concern. Gender disparities have been widely observed in other surgical procedures such as coronary artery bypass grafting.[63,64] Early data regarding PN abstracted from NIS data from 1988 to 2002 showed that only 6.7% of women underwent PN versus 8.0% of men (P<.0001).[4] More contemporary data abstracted from the SEER database between 1999 and 2006 found that men were still 22% more likely to undergo PN compared with women. This disparity persisted even in a separate logistical model that included age, indicating that the bias was not limited to a specific age category.[52] Even when controlling for various other risk factors such as tumor size, year of surgery, age, marital status, and place of SEER registry, gender has been shown to be a statistically significant risk factor predicting use of RN over PN.[55] This finding has been reported in European populations as well.[51,59] This observation is particularly concerning because women are more likely to be overtreated with RN given the greater likelihood of their being diagnosed with a benign tumor compared with men.[52,65,66]

There may be many contributing reasons as to why this gender disparity exists both in the United States and internationally. One proposed theory attributes the disparity to physician bias, because it has been postulated that physicians may underestimate the risk of CKD in women based on their lower baseline serum creatinine levels. This error may be further compounded by the belief that women generally have fewer comorbid conditions and thus may accrue less overall benefit from the selection of PN, which is often considered to be a riskier and more technically demanding procedure. Alternatively, patient preference to undergo

a more conservative procedure could be a second reasonable explanation. It has been similarly postulated that women may prefer a more definitive procedure to minimize the risk of recurrence. Finally, it is also conceivable that women may more frequently elect to undergo active surveillance on the basis that they are 2 to 4 times more likely to have benign or complex cystic renal tumors compared with men.[52,65,66] However, although any or all of these factors may apply, the true causes of this gender bias in the usage of PN have not been adequately explained.

Patient comorbidities

The increased presence of comorbidities has been shown to reduce the likelihood of undergoing PN. Analysis of early NIS data showed that patients with a Charlson score of greater than 3 were found to be 60% less likely to undergo PN than those with scores of 0 to 2 between 1988 and 2001.[4] In a more contemporary series encompassing NIS data from 2003 to 2008, those with an Elixhauser index of 2 to 3 or greater than 3 were found to be 83% and 67%, respectively, less likely to undergo PN compared with those with a score of 0 to 1.[54] This trend has been reported in the European population as well; Fedeli and colleagues[59] reported that patients with a Charlson comorbidity index 1 or greater were significantly less likely to undergo PN compared with counterparts with Charlson index 0 on both single and multivariate analysis.

Although at face value, the selection of RN in sicker patients in an attempt to avoid a higher rate of perioperative morbidity and complications may seem reasonable, it could be conversely argued that this population of patients with a greater number of comorbidities has the most to gain from a nephron-sparing approach with respect to their long-term renal, cardiovascular, and survival outcomes. Furthermore, even if PN could not be pursued secondary to a patient's extensive comorbidities, it stands to reason that active surveillance rather than RN may offer better long-term outcomes. The ideal rate of PN in populations with extensive comorbidities remains unknown.

Other patient demographic factors

Race has been shown to be an independent predictor of PN usage as well in some population-based cohort studies. NIS data abstracted from 1988 to 2001 showed that blacks and Hispanics were more likely to undergo PN than the reference race of whites.[4] Using more recent NIS data, Kim and colleagues[54] recently reported that blacks still had statistically significant higher odds of undergoing PN compared with whites (OR 1.11,

$P = .02$). However, this finding may represent the influence of an alternate confounding risk factor because there have been reports of no significant disparity between race on some multivariate analyses of contemporary SEER data.[52,55]

There have been numerous other disparities in the usage of PN identified by various investigators from various patient demographic factors. Different studies have suggested that those with private insurance,[54,58] who are married[53] and undergoing elective[4,54] (as opposed to emergent) resection are more likely to undergo PN for renal lesions. However, long-term trends investigating the application of PN to these patient populations have not been nearly as thoroughly examined as those regarding age, race, gender, and the presence of comorbidities.

Hospital and surgeon characteristics

The use of PN may vary by some hospital-level factors as well. It has been reported that patients treated at teaching hospitals may be more likely to undergo PN compared with those treated at nonteaching hospitals. Using NIS data from between 1988 and 2002, Hollenbeck and colleagues[4] reported that the PN rate at teaching hospitals was 10.5% versus only 5.2% at nonteaching hospitals ($P<.0001$). When restricting the analysis only to NIS data from 1998 to 2002, Porter and colleagues[58] found that those treated in teaching hospitals were still nearly twice as likely to undergo PN compared with the referent group treated at nonteaching hospitals (OR 1.95, $P<.001$). This trend has persisted even in the most contemporary of series; Kim and colleagues,[54] using NIS data from between 2003 and 2008, reported that patients treated at teaching hospitals were still 1.3 times more likely to undergo PN compared with those treated at nonteaching hospitals (OR 1.31, $P<.001$).

A similar increased likelihood of undergoing PN has been witnessed in urban settings. Analysis of NIS data from 1998 to 2002 led to the conclusion that those treated in urban settings had a marginally higher likelihood of undergoing PN than their rural counterparts.[4] Analysis of the more recent NIS data from 2003 to 2008 revealed that this disparity has not improved, because those treated in urban hospitals were still more likely to undergo PN (OR 1.13, $P = .05$).[54] It was also noted that patients treated at hospitals located in the northeast were significantly more likely to undergo PN compared with those treated in the midwest (OR 0.76), south (OR 0.76), or west (OR 0.75) United States. Kim and colleagues[54] also reported that patients treated in hospitals located in ZIP (zone improvement plan) codes with median household

annual income exceeding $63,000 were significantly more likely to undergo PN compared with their counterparts treated in ZIP codes with median annual income less than $39,000. The question of which of the hospital region-oriented characteristics has the strongest effect on likelihood of PN remains unknown.

Hospital nephrectomy volume has also been shown to be an independent predictor of the frequency of PN utilization by some population-based cohort studies. From NIS data from 1988 to 2002, Hollenbeck and colleagues[4] reported that the patients treated at hospitals with annual nephrectomy volume greater than or equal to 28 were 2.5 times more likely to undergo PN compared with patients treated at very-low-volume hospitals (annual volume 1–5). A similarly significant trend showing increasing use of PN with increasing annual nephrectomy volume was also seen in hospitals with volume 17 to 27 (OR 1.7), 11 to 16 (OR 1.2), and 6 to 10 (OR 1.1) compared with a referent very-low-volume group. This trend toward an increased likelihood of PN at higher-volume nephrectomy centers was confirmed in studies based on NIS data from 1998 to 2002 and from 2003 to 2008.[54,58] A similar disparity in PN rate between hospitals by nephrectomy volume has been observed in European populations as well.[59] Although the observation that PN is more likely at high-nephrectomy-volume hospitals is unmistakable, it is not known whether this is the result of a high rate of referrals of PN patients to high-volume centers or the inappropriate use of RN at low-volume centers. More research on this topic is required to answer this question.

Differences in surgeon characteristics are likely to play a role in the determination of whether PN is used in the treatment of a renal mass. Miller and colleagues[40] reported that proportion of variance in use of PN due to surgeon-level determinants was greater than for any other factor except for tumor size. One example of a surgeon-related characteristic that may affect the rate of PN utilization is annual surgeon nephrectomy volume. When Porter and Lin[58] analyzed NIS data from 1998 to 2002 by stratifying patients into quartiles based on the operating surgeon's nephrectomy volume, they found a statistically significant increase in PN usage with each progressive increase in quartile. Similar to the discussion regarding the data surrounding variations in PN usage between hospitals with varying nephrectomy volumes, it is unknown whether this trend represents a high rate of referrals of PN candidates to higher-volume surgeons or the inappropriate usage of RN by low-volume nephrectomists.

International trends

Similar trends have been observed internationally as well. For example, from data extracted from England's Hospital Episode Statistics database, Nuttall and colleagues[67] found that PN was performed in less than 5% of surgeries for renal malignancies in 2000 to 2001. The European rate of adoption in the 10 years since then has been similarly sluggish. Using a regional archive of hospital discharge records from the Veneto region of northeastern Italy, Fedeli and colleagues[59] reported that the usage of PN increased over the course of their study from being used in 22% of all oncologic kidney surgeries in 1999 to 31% in 2007. However, as has been described in the US literature, European tertiary-care centers have been quicker to use PN. Zini and colleagues,[51] after analyzing data regarding all T1-T2N0M0 tumors from 6 European tertiary-care centers, reported that the overall PN rate increased from 11.2% between 1987 and 1991 to 37.4% from 2000 to 2003. Between 2004 and 2007, the PN rate surpassed that of RN in these tertiary-care centers, reaching 50.1%. When stratified into groups defined by tumor size less than 2 cm, tumor size between 2.1 and 4 cm, and tumor size between 4.1 and 7 cm, the investigators reported PN rates between 2004 and 2007 of 86.3%, 69.3%, and 35.3%, respectively. Although there have been single-institution reports of US tertiary-care centers with PN rates of up to 90% for small T1a tumors and 60% for T1b tumors,[50] large population-based cohort studies have consistently indicated a lower and more slowly increasing PN rate nationwide.

The effect of laparoscopy on the adoption of PN

It has been suggested that the widespread acceptance of laparoscopy has contributed to the underuse of PN for small renal masses. This conjecture is based on the premise that technical rigors and perioperative risk associated with performing laparoscopic PN (LPN) has left many urologists with the choice of choosing between a minimally invasive or a nephron-sparing surgical approach to renal masses (ie, LRN vs OPN). Although this question has been investigated by some population-based cohort studies, the results have been conflicting. Using the population-based Ontario cancer registry, Abouassaly and colleagues[68] found that the odds of PN increased by 18% per year until January 2003 and subsequently decreased by 12% per year. They consequently concluded that the introduction of LRN coincided with decreased use and adoption of PN. By contrast, Perotti and colleagues, after retrospectively analyzing their database of patients with T1 renal masses, concluded that laparoscopy did not seem to result in an underuse of PN.

MINIMALLY INVASIVE PN

Although most newly diagnosed renal masses are amenable to removal with LPN, its widespread adoption has likely been limited by its technical difficulty and an increased risk in significant complications. A recent article[40] estimated its use at only 3% of all RCC cases nationally.

An association between era of training and the use of laparoscopy has been reported in the literature. Filson and colleagues[36] reported that more recent medical school graduates (1991 or after) were more likely to use laparoscopy in the management of renal masses than earlier trained counterparts. Furthermore, this disparity seems to apply to the usage of laparoscopy within all of urology (not just among nephrectomists), because a recent study based on questionnaires found a correlation between younger urologists and those who practiced laparoscopy as a primary surgeon.[69] A reasonable explanation for this may be that urologists who graduated after 1991 are more likely to have been exposed to laparoscopy during their residency and thus to have undergone some degree of formal laparoscopic training. This explanation suggests that formal laparoscopic training may be necessary to overcome a steep learning curve associated with laparoscopic surgery. In 2004, Hollenbeck and colleagues[70] reported that clinically significant improvements in laparoscopic skills can be realized with participation in as few as 13 procedures or serving as a surgeon in 6 procedures. This finding has led to the proposal that a minifellowship postgraduate training model be used, through which practicing urologists could exercise and perfect their skills with the aid of a laparoscopic mentor, to master the skill required to safely perform LPN.[71]

The recent development of robotic-assisted LPN may help bridge this gap by enabling more urologists to perform LPN.[1] There have been several retrospective, single-institutional studies showing comparable oncologic outcomes and favorable perioperative parameters such as warm ischemia time, estimated blood loss, and complication rate.[72–74] However, no large-scale population-based studies exist that examine trends in the use of robotic-assisted LPN.

TRENDS IN THE USE OF ABLATIVE THERAPIES

The increased technical demands associated with PN have led to interest in other NSS techniques that may be more easily adopted by practicing urologists and that may present less potential morbidity and risk to patients. One proposed alternative is the use of thermoablation in the treatment of small renal masses. This form of NSS is being increasingly offered by academic institutions throughout the country. A recent survey-based study found that ablation was offered by 93% of responding academic urology centers. Cryoablation was used more frequently than radiofrequency ablation (RFA) (79% vs 55%). Based on survey responses to hypothetical case scenarios, it was further observed that in young healthy patients, an extirpative approach was still recommended, namely LPN for small peripheral masses (90%). LRN, and not open PN, was recommended for small hilar masses (67%). By contrast, ablation was recommended for an anteriorly located peripheral renal mass in an elderly patient with comorbidities (53%).[75]

A population-based study performed on data abstracted from 2004 to 2007 SEER data regarding patients who underwent a procedure for a renal tumor 7 cm or less in size was published by Choueiri and colleagues[76] in 2011. These investigators reported that there were 578 instances of thermal ablation (TA) among the 15,145 patients who underwent a procedure for organ-confined RCC T1 tumors between 2004 and 2007. On multivariable analysis, it was determined that increasing age, decreasing tumor size (<4 cm), and lower education (no college degree) were all predictors of TA use over PN or RN. Furthermore, as seen with both LRN and PN, more recent year of diagnosis (analyzed as a continuous variable) was also a significant predictor of TA over PN or RN, suggesting increased adoption with time.[76] Although some single-institution series have reported good oncologic outcomes after ablative techniques,[77,78] a recent meta-analysis reported a significantly higher rate of recurrence in patients treated with both cryoablation and RFA (relative risk [RR] 7.45 and 18.23, respectively, $P<.001$) compared with those treated with PN even at mean follow-up of only 47.1 months.[79] The widespread acceptance of these techniques is even further limited by a general lack of long-term data regarding efficacy. However, these shortcomings aside, cryoablation and RFA can potentially combine the relative advantages of nephron-sparing and minimally invasive approaches to renal masses without the technical considerations of LPN. For this reason, thermal-based tissue-ablative techniques represent an emerging and appealing option for patients with small renal masses.

TRENDS IN THE USE OF ACTIVE SURVEILLANCE

The current literature investigating the use of active surveillance for management of small renal tumors is largely composed of small, single-institution, retrospective studies. Although there are some ongoing trials investigating the use of observation nationwide, there are no large population-based cohort studies assessing trends in the use of active surveillance for small, incidentally found, renal tumors. Nevertheless, we anticipate that the use of active surveillance will increase, particularly in those patients with extensive comorbidities whose overall survival is unlikely to be affected by a small incidentally found renal mass. The optimal usage of active surveillance is discussed further elsewhere in this issue by Kim and colleagues.

SUMMARY

Over the last 20 years, there has been an increase in the incidence of renal tumors, with the greatest increase seen in incidental small renal masses, resulting in a downward size and stage migration. These changes in the landscape of renal tumors have brought about a paradigm shift in the management of these masses such that NSS, minimally invasive techniques, and active surveillance are frequently considered preferable to the previous gold standard, ORN. Despite adoption of many of the advances in the surgical management of kidney cancer at tertiary centers, population-based cohort studies indicate that there continue to be significant disparities in the delivery of care across the country. Further investigation is required to determine the barriers to diffusion of new techniques and technology as well as to ensure equal access to quality care in the United States.

REFERENCES

1. Chen DY, Uzzo RG. Optimal management of localized renal cell carcinoma: surgery, ablation, or active surveillance. J Natl Compr Canc Netw 2009; 7(6):635–42 [quiz: 643].
2. Jemal A, Siegel R, Xu J, et al. Cancer statistics, 2010. CA Cancer J Clin 2010;60(5):277–300.
3. Hollingsworth JM, Miller DC, Daignault S, et al. Rising incidence of small renal masses: a need to reassess treatment effect. J Natl Cancer Inst 2006; 98(18):1331–4.
4. Hollenbeck BK, Taub DA, Miller DC, et al. National utilization trends of partial nephrectomy for renal cell carcinoma: a case of underutilization? Urology 2006;67(2):254–9.

5. Mindrup SR, Pierre JS, Dahmoush L, et al. The prevalence of renal cell carcinoma diagnosed at autopsy. BJU Int 2005;95(1):31–3.

6. Chow WH, Devesa SS, Warren JL, et al. Rising incidence of renal cell cancer in the United States. JAMA 1999;281(17):1628–31.

7. Kutikov A, Fossett LK, Ramchandani P, et al. Incidence of benign pathologic findings at partial nephrectomy for solitary renal mass presumed to be renal cell carcinoma on preoperative imaging. Urology 2006;68(4):737–40.

8. Snyder ME, Bach A, Kattan MW, et al. Incidence of benign lesions for clinically localized renal masses smaller than 7 cm in radiological diameter: influence of sex. J Urol 2006;176(6 Pt 1):2391–5 [discussion: 2395–6].

9. Pahernik S, Ziegler S, Roos F, et al. Small renal tumors: correlation of clinical and pathological features with tumor size. J Urol 2007;178(2):414–7 [discussion: 416–7].

10. Remzi M, Ozsoy M, Klingler HC, et al. Are small renal tumors harmless? Analysis of histopathological features according to tumors 4 cm or less in diameter. J Urol 2006;176(3):896–9.

11. Robson CJ. Radical nephrectomy for renal cell carcinoma. J Urol 1963;89:37–42.

12. Clayman RV, Kavoussi LR, Soper NJ, et al. Laparoscopic nephrectomy: initial case report. J Urol 1991;146(2):278–82.

13. Wolf JS Jr, Merion RM, Leichtman AB, et al. Randomized controlled trial of hand-assisted laparoscopic versus open surgical live donor nephrectomy. Transplantation 2001;72(2):284–90.

14. Simforoosh N, Basiri A, Tabibi A, et al. Comparison of laparoscopic and open donor nephrectomy: a randomized controlled trial. BJU Int 2005;95(6):851–5.

15. Oyen O, Andersen M, Mathisen L, et al. Laparoscopic versus open living-donor nephrectomy: experiences from a prospective, randomized, single-center study focusing on donor safety. Transplantation 2005;79(9):1236–40.

16. Dunn MD, Portis AJ, Shalhav AL, et al. Laparoscopic versus open radical nephrectomy: a 9-year experience. J Urol 2000;164(4):1153–9.

17. McDougall E, Clayman RV, Elashry OM. Laparoscopic radical nephrectomy for renal tumor: the Washington University experience. J Urol 1996;155(4):1180–5.

18. Eskicorapci SY, Teber D, Schulze M, et al. Laparoscopic radical nephrectomy: the new gold standard surgical treatment for localized renal cell carcinoma. ScientificWorldJournal 2007;7:825–36.

19. Novick AC. Renal-sparing surgery for renal cell carcinoma. Urol Clin North Am 1993;20(2):277–82.

20. Uzzo RG, Novick AC. Nephron sparing surgery for renal tumors: indications, techniques and outcomes. J Urol 2001;166(1):6–18.

21. Huang WC, Levey AS, Serio AM, et al. Chronic kidney disease after nephrectomy in patients with renal cortical tumours: a retrospective cohort study. Lancet Oncol 2006;7(9):735–40.

22. Lee CT, Katz J, Shi W, et al. Surgical management of renal tumors 4 cm. or less in a contemporary cohort. J Urol 2000;163(3):730–6.

23. Dash A, Vickers AJ, Schachter LR, et al. Comparison of outcomes in elective partial vs radical nephrectomy for clear cell renal cell carcinoma of 4-7 cm. BJU Int 2006;97(5):939–45.

24. Leibovich BC, Blute ML, Cheville JC, et al. Nephron sparing surgery for appropriately selected renal cell carcinoma between 4 and 7 cm results in outcome similar to radical nephrectomy. J Urol 2004;171(3):1066–70.

25. Patard JJ, Shvarts O, Lam JS, et al. Safety and efficacy of partial nephrectomy for all T1 tumors based on an international multicenter experience. J Urol 2004;171(6 Pt 1):2181–5 [quiz: 2435].

26. Deane LA, Clayman RV. Review of minimally invasive renal therapies: needle-based and extracorporeal. Urology 2006;68(Suppl 1):26–37.

27. Hui GC, Tuncali K, Tatli S, et al. Comparison of percutaneous and surgical approaches to renal tumor ablation: metaanalysis of effectiveness and complication rates. J Vasc Interv Radiol 2008;19(9):1311–20.

28. Lucas SM, Stern JM, Adibi M, et al. Renal function outcomes in patients treated for renal masses smaller than 4 cm by ablative and extirpative techniques. J Urol 2008;179(1):75–9 [discussion: 79–80].

29. Chawla SN, Crispen PL, Hanlon AL, et al. The natural history of observed enhancing renal masses: meta-analysis and review of the world literature. J Urol 2006;175(2):425–31.

30. Ono Y, Kinukawa T, Hattori R, et al. The long-term outcome of laparoscopic radical nephrectomy for small renal cell carcinoma. J Urol 2001;165(6 Pt 1):1867–70.

31. Chan DY, Caddedu JA, Jarrett TW, et al. Laparoscopic radical nephrectomy: cancer control for renal cell carcinoma. J Urol 2001;166(6):2095–9 [discussion: 2099–100].

32. Gill IS, Meraney AM, Schweizer DK, et al. Laparoscopic radical nephrectomy in 100 patients: a single center experience from the United States. Cancer 2001;92(7):1843–55.

33. Janetschek G, Jeschke K, Peschel R, et al. Laparoscopic surgery for stage T1 renal cell carcinoma: radical nephrectomy and wedge resection. Eur Urol 2000;38(2):131–8.

34. Permpongkosol S, Chan DY, Link RE, et al. Long-term survival analysis after laparoscopic radical nephrectomy. J Urol 2005;174(4 Pt 1):1222–5.

35. Miller DC, Taub DA, Dunn RL, et al. Laparoscopy for renal cell carcinoma: diffusion versus regionalization? J Urol 2006;176(3):1102–6 [discussion: 1106–7].

36. Filson CP, Banerjee M, Wolf JS Jr, et al. Surgeon characteristics and long-term trends in the adoption of laparoscopic radical nephrectomy. J Urol 2011; 185(6):2072–7.

37. Finlayson SR, Laycock WS, Birkmeyer JD. National trends in utilization and outcomes of antireflux surgery. Surg Endosc 2003;17(6):864–7.

38. Fendrick AM, Escarce JJ, McLane C, et al. Hospital adoption of laparoscopic cholecystectomy. Med Care 1994;32(10):1058–63.

39. Best S, Ercole B, Lee C, et al. Minimally invasive therapy for renal cell carcinoma: is there a new community standard? Urology 2004;64(1):22–5.

40. Miller DC, Saigal CS, Banerjee M, et al. Diffusion of surgical innovation among patients with kidney cancer. Cancer 2008;112(8):1708–17.

41. Campbell SC, Novick AC, Belldegrun A, et al. Guideline for management of the clinical T1 renal mass. J Urol 2009;182(4):1271–9.

42. Becker F, Siemer S, Hack M, et al. Excellent long-term cancer control with elective nephron-sparing surgery for selected renal cell carcinomas measuring more than 4 cm. Eur Urol 2006;49(6):1058–63 [discussion: 1063–4].

43. Becker F, Siemer S, Humke U, et al. Elective nephron sparing surgery should become standard treatment for small unilateral renal cell carcinoma: long-term survival data of 216 patients. Eur Urol 2006;49(2):308–13.

44. Thompson RH, Siddiqui S, Lohse CM, et al, Siddiqui S, Lohse CM. Partial versus radical nephrectomy for 4 to 7 cm renal cortical tumors. J Urol 2009;182(6):2601–6.

45. Stiles KP, Moffatt MJ, Agodoa LY, et al. Renal cell carcinoma as a cause of end-stage renal disease in the United States: patient characteristics and survival. Kidney Int 2003;64(1):247–53.

46. McKiernan J, Yossepowitch O, Kattan MW, et al. Partial nephrectomy for renal cortical tumors: pathologic findings and impact on outcome. Urology 2002;60(6):1003–9.

47. Lau WK, Blute ML, Weaver AL, et al. Matched comparison of radical nephrectomy vs nephron-sparing surgery in patients with unilateral renal cell carcinoma and a normal contralateral kidney. Mayo Clin Proc 2000;75(12):1236–42.

48. Go AS, Chertow GM, Fan D, et al. Chronic kidney disease and the risks of death, cardiovascular events, and hospitalization. N Engl J Med 2004; 351(13):1296–305.

49. Rifkin DE, Shlipak MG, Katz R, et al. Rapid kidney function decline and mortality risk in older adults. Arch Intern Med 2008;168(20):2212–8.

50. Thompson RH, Kaag M, Vickers A, et al. Contemporary use of partial nephrectomy at a tertiary care center in the United States. J Urol 2009;181(3): 993–7.

51. Zini L, Patard JJ, Capitanio U, et al. The use of partial nephrectomy in European tertiary care centers. Eur J Surg Oncol 2009;35(6):636–42.

52. Dulabon LM, Lowrance WT, Russo P, et al. Trends in renal tumor surgery delivery within the United States. Cancer 2010;116(10):2316–21.

53. Miller DC, Hollingsworth JM, Hafez KS, et al. Partial nephrectomy for small renal masses: an emerging quality of care concern? J Urol 2006;175(3 Pt 1): 853–7 [discussion: 858].

54. Kim SP, Shah ND, Weight CJ, et al. Contemporary trends in nephrectomy for renal cell carcinoma in the United States: results from a population based cohort. J Urol 2011;186(5):1779–85.

55. Baillargeon-Gagne S, Jeldres C, Lughezzani G, et al. A comparative population-based analysis of the rate of partial vs radical nephrectomy for clinically localized renal cell carcinoma. BJU Int 2010; 105(3):359–64.

56. Broughton GJ, Clark PE, Barocas DA, et al. Tumour size, tumour complexity, and surgical approach are associated with nephrectomy type in small renal cortical tumours treated electively. BJU Int 2011. [Epub ahead of print].

57. Satasivam P, Rajarubendra N, Chia PH, et al. Trends in the use of nephron-sparing surgery (NSS) at an Australian tertiary referral centre: an analysis of surgical decision-making using the R.E.N.A.L. nephrometry scoring system. BJU Int 2011. [Epub ahead of print].

58. Porter MP, Lin DW. Trends in renal cancer surgery and patient provider characteristics associated with partial nephrectomy in the United States. Urol Oncol 2007;25(4):298–302.

59. Fedeli U, Novara G, Alba N, et al. Trends from 1999 to 2007 in the surgical treatments of kidney cancer in Europe: data from the Veneto Region, Italy. BJU Int 2010;105(9):1255–9.

60. Van Poppel H, Da Pozzo L, Albrecht W, et al. A prospective randomized EORTC intergroup phase 3 study comparing the complications of elective nephron-sparing surgery and radical nephrectomy for low-stage renal cell carcinoma. Eur Urol 2007; 51(6):1606–15.

61. Stephenson AJ, Hakimi AA, Snyder ME, et al. Complications of radical and partial nephrectomy in a large contemporary cohort. J Urol 2004; 171(1):130–4.

62. Huang WC, Elkin EB, Levey AS, et al. Partial nephrectomy versus radical nephrectomy in patients with small renal tumors–is there a difference in mortality and cardiovascular outcomes? J Urol 2009;181(1):55–61 [discussion: 61–2].

63. Ayanian JZ, Epstein AM. Differences in the use of procedures between women and men hospitalized for coronary heart disease. N Engl J Med 1991; 325(4):221–5.

64. Healy B. The Yentl syndrome. N Engl J Med 1991; 325(4):274–6.

65. Eggener SE, Rubenstein JN, Smith ND, et al. Renal tumors in young adults. J Urol 2004;171(1):106–10.

66. Murphy AM, Buck AM, Benson MC, et al. Increasing detection rate of benign renal tumors: evaluation of factors predicting for benign tumor histologic features during past two decades. Urology 2009; 73(6):1293–7.

67. Nuttall M, Cathcart P, van der Meulen J, et al. A description of radical nephrectomy practice and outcomes in England: 1995-2002. BJU Int 2005; 96(1):58–61.

68. Abouassaly R, Alibhai SM, Tomlinson G, et al. Unintended consequences of laparoscopic surgery on partial nephrectomy for kidney cancer. J Urol 2010; 183(2):467–72.

69. Abdelshehid CS, Eichel L, Lee D, et al. Current trends in urologic laparoscopic surgery. J Endourol 2005;19(1):15–20.

70. Hollenbeck BK, Seifman BD, Wolf JS Jr. Clinical skills acquisition for hand-assisted laparoscopic donor nephrectomy. J Urol 2004;171(1):35–9.

71. Shalhav AL, Dabagia MD, Wagner TT, et al. Training postgraduate urologists in laparoscopic surgery: the current challenge. J Urol 2002;167(5):2135–7.

72. Gupta GN, Boris R, Chung P, et al. Robot-assisted laparoscopic partial nephrectomy for tumors greater than 4 cm and high nephrometry score: feasibility, renal functional, and oncological outcomes with minimum 1 year follow-up. Urol Oncol 2011. [Epub ahead of print].

73. Deane LA, Lee HJ, Box GN, et al. Robotic versus standard laparoscopic partial/wedge nephrectomy: a comparison of intraoperative and perioperative results from a single institution. J Endourol 2008;22(5):947–52.

74. Benway BM, Bhayani SB, Rogers CG, et al. Robot assisted partial nephrectomy versus laparoscopic partial nephrectomy for renal tumors: a multi-institutional analysis of perioperative outcomes. J Urol 2009;182(3):866–72.

75. Bandi G, Hedican SP, Nakada SY. Current practice patterns in the use of ablation technology for the management of small renal masses at academic centers in the United States. Urology 2008;71(1): 113–7.

76. Choueiri TK, Schutz FA, Hevelone ND, et al. Thermal ablation vs surgery for localized kidney cancer: a Surveillance, Epidemiology, and End Results (SEER) database analysis. Urology 2011;78(1):93–8.

77. McDougal WS, Gervais D, McGovern F, et al. Long-term followup of patients with renal cell carcinoma treated with radio frequency ablation with curative intent. J Urol 2005;174(1):61–3.

78. Levinson A, Su L-M, Agarwal D, et al. Long-term oncological and overall outcomes of percutaneous radio frequency ablation in high risk surgical patients with a solitary small renal mass. J Urol 2008;180(2):499–504.

79. Kunkle DA, Egleston BL, Uzzo RG. Excise, ablate or observe: the small renal mass dilemma–a meta-analysis and review. J Urol 2008;179(4):1227–33 [discussion: 1233–4].

Contemporary Imaging of the Renal Mass

Stella K. Kang, MD[a], Hersh Chandarana, MD[b],*

KEYWORDS
- Renal mass • Ultrasonography • CT • MRI
- Dual-energy CT • Diffusion-weighted imaging

Most renal masses are discovered incidentally on medical imaging.[1,2] Although approximately 80% of all renal lesions are malignant,[3] up to 38% of masses with diameters less than 1 cm are benign.[4] Increased detection of renal masses has prompted the need for improved characterization as well as exploration of less invasive treatment strategies. Ultrasonography, computed tomography (CT), and magnetic resonance imaging (MRI) are currently available imaging modalities used to evaluate renal masses. Understanding the strengths and limitations of these modalities can enable better use of these resources and has important implications in the management of patients with renal tumors. In addition, advanced MRI techniques can potentially provide information beyond anatomic description of tumors and may assist in noninvasive assessment of renal cell cancer (RCC) aggressiveness.

ULTRASONOGRAPHY

Major advantages of sonographic evaluation include low cost and lack of ionizing radiation or need for intravenous contrast administration. The modality is widely accessible and is therefore commonly used for initial screening evaluation of renal disease or lesions. It is also routinely used to discriminate cystic lesions from solid lesions, monitor growth of a lesion, and evaluate hyperdense lesions found on CT that could be cysts.[5] Cystic lesions are examined for the presence of internal septations, calcifications, vascularity, and mural nodularity. Presence of these features increases the likelihood of a lesion being

malignant, thus requiring definitive characterization with a dedicated renal CT or MRI.[6] Although recent studies suggest that use of contrast-enhanced ultrasonography has the potential to improve detection and characterization of renal lesions,[7] these contrast agents are not approved by the Federal Drug Administration (FDA), and are not available for clinical use in the United States.

One of the limitations of the sonography is the lower accuracy for smaller lesions compared with CT. In a study by Jamis-Dow and colleagues,[8] ultrasonography detected 58% of lesions sized 15 to 20 mm, compared with CT, which detected all the (100%) lesions. Characterization of renal masses on ultrasonography is also limited because of the variable echogenicity of RCC, which can range from hypoechoic to hyperechoic when compared with the renal parenchyma. Solid hyperechoic RCC (**Fig. 1**) may overlap in appearance with benign angiomyolipomas.[9] Furthermore, ultrasonography is user dependent, which can lead to interobserver variability in follow-up of lesions and in size measurements.

CT

CT is currently the modality of choice for characterization and staging of renal masses. CT is more than 90% sensitive for detecting small renal masses.[8] Multidetector CT (MDCT), the most recent generation of scanners, is now in widespread use and uses multiple rows of detectors providing nearly isotropic datasets. Images can therefore be reformatted in coronal or sagittal

[a] Department of Radiology, New York University Langone Medical Center, 462 First Avenue, NBV 3W39, New York, NY 10016, USA
[b] Department of Radiology, New York University Langone Medical Center, 560 First Avenue, New York, NY 10016, USA
* Corresponding author.
E-mail address: Hersh.chandarana@nyumc.org

Urol Clin N Am 39 (2012) 161–170
doi:10.1016/j.ucl.2012.01.002

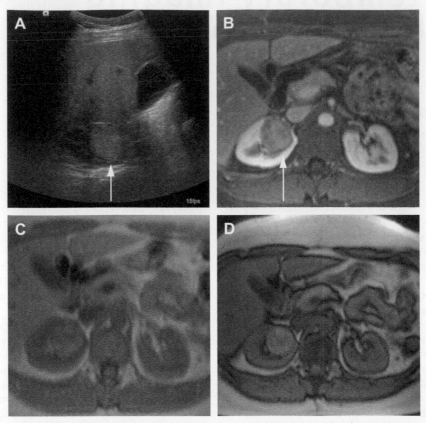

Fig. 1. (*A*) Ultrasonography of the right upper quadrant shows right kidney with echogenic mass, which may be seen with angiomyolipoma, but RCC may be echogenic in appearance. (*B*) Contrast-enhanced T1 3D fat-suppressed image demonstrates enhancement. There is no evidence of India ink artifact or intravoxel fat on (*C*) T1 in-phase and (*D*) out-of-phase images to suggest angiomyolipoma. An atypical oncocytic neoplasm was diagnosed on surgical pathologic examination.

planes with near-equal resolution. The MDCT protocol for renal mass evaluation includes a noncontrast phase followed by postcontrast acquisitions acquired at multiple times after injection of contrast, with corticomedullary, nephrographic, and delayed phases of enhancement at approximately 40 seconds, 90 seconds, and 7 minutes after contrast injection, respectively. The nephrographic phase serves best for assessing the presence of a renal lesion and its enhancement and is thus sufficient for detection and characterization of renal lesions. Corticomedullary (arterial) and urographic phases are often acquired to provide additional valuable information for presurgical planning and assessing proximity or involvement of the collecting system (**Fig. 2**). An important drawback to this multiphase technique is the higher ionizing radiation dose to the patient.

Assessment of Renal Lesions

The presence of enhancement is the most important factor in determining the likelihood of

malignancy in a renal mass. Enhancement on CT is defined as an attenuation increase of at least 15 to 20 Hounsfield units (HU) on postcontrast image with respect to the noncontrast acquisition. Lesions demonstrating an increase of up to 10 HU are not categorized as enhancing masses because of the phenomenon of pseudoenhancement, which causes a renal cyst to appear increased in density on contrast-enhanced images.[6] In cases in which a lesion is incompletely characterized because of increase in attenuation between 10 and 20 HU on postcontrast CT, MRI may be helpful as a problem-solving tool. MRI can also be useful in the assessment of hypovascular malignancies such as papillary RCC, which may be mistaken for renal cysts on a postcontrast CT in nephrographic phase due to low level of enhancement.

Studies have reported the possibility of differentiating papillary type RCCs from other subtypes on CT using the degree of contrast enhancement. In one study, attenuation of less than 100 HU on the corticomedullary phase of enhancement was 95.7% accurate for distinguishing papillary

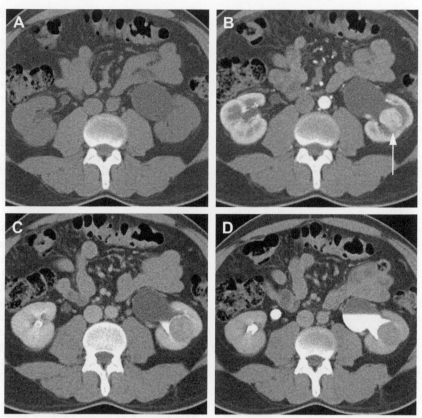

Fig. 2. Multiphase CT performed for renal mass evaluation. (*A*) Noncontrast and (*B*) arterial phase images reveal an endophytic enhancing left renal mass in this patient with a history of ureteropelvic junction obstruction. (*C*) Nephrographic and (*D*) urographic phases demonstrate splaying of the calyces by this interpolar endophytic mass.

carcinomas from clear cell carcinomas after normalizing for the degree of aortic enhancement.[10] A homogeneous pattern of enhancement has also been reported to be significantly associated with papillary RCC.[11,12]

Cystic lesions

The Bosniak classification system is both an imaging and clinical management system for evaluation of cystic renal lesions. Although this classification scheme was initially described based on the findings at CT, it is also applicable to MRI.[13] Category 1 lesions are simple cysts, category 2 lesions are mildly complicated benign cysts, and category 4 lesions are cystic renal neoplasms or cystic RCC. Diagnosis and management of these lesions is straight forward, such that category 1 and 2 lesions are benign and no further workup is required, whereas category 4 lesions are managed surgically. Category 2F lesions are moderately complicated cystic masses that are indeterminate and require follow-up to demonstrate stability and exclude malignancy. Category 3 lesions have some features that can be seen

with cystic RCC, and, because of suspicion of malignancy, these lesions are managed surgically.

Although CT remains the modality of choice in evaluation of renal lesions, some of the disadvantages of CT include limited characterization of lesions less than 1 cm in diameter, the potential for allergic reaction or nephrotoxicity due to the iodinated contrast medium, and exposure to ionizing radiation, which is of concern in patients undergoing repeated CT examinations.

DUAL-ENERGY CT

The recent development of dual-energy CT (DECT) technology has the potential to lower radiation dose to the patient. DECT involves simultaneous acquisition of CT data at 2 different energies or peak tube voltages.[14] Different materials (such as iodine and soft tissue) demonstrate unique attenuation differences at the varying tube voltages, allowing for material decomposition. When the technology is applied to remove iodine contribution from a postcontrast image, the generated set of images is termed virtual noncontrast dataset.

Use of the virtual noncontrast dataset has been studied as a replacement for a true noncontrast acquisition in the evaluation of renal lesions. The single-phase DECT examination resulted in a 47% reduction in radiation dose compared with a dual-phase CT examination in a study by Graser and colleagues,[15] while preserving accurate lesion characterization. Review of a single-phase postcontrast DECT examination in conjunction with virtual noncontrast data set produced an accuracy of 94.6% in diagnosing malignant renal lesions, when compared with 96% accuracy using a 2-phase CT examination with a true noncontrast data set. Alternatively it is possible to measure iodine concentration (instead of attenuation values) within the lesion.[16] Enhancing renal mass demonstrates presence of iodine, whereas benign nonenhancing lesion has absence of intralesional iodine (**Fig. 3**). Although preliminary results of renal mass evaluation with DECT are encouraging, the technology is not yet widely available and clinical use is in early stages.

MRI

MRI can be a potent problem-solving tool in clinical practice for characterization of renal masses. Like CT, MRI offers accurate anatomic information in evaluation of renal lesion. However, unlike CT, advanced MRI techniques can provide information about tissue structure and function without exposure to ionizing radiation. MRI also serves as an alternative to CT in patients with allergies to iodinated contrast.

MRI of the kidneys is usually performed on 1.5- or 3-T magnets, which are widely available. Recent advances in MRI hardware and software enable faster imaging so that sequences through the

kidneys can be acquired in a breath-hold (suspended respiratory motion) with an examination time of approximately 30 minutes. Free-breathing techniques are also in development[17] and may be useful in subjects who are unable to suspend respiration. The standard MRI protocol for renal mass evaluation includes multiple sequences (**Table 1**): T2-weighted imaging, T1-weighted opposed-phase imaging (with in-phase and out-of-phase sequences) for detection of microscopic fat, and fat-suppressed T1-weighted gradient-echo acquisition before and after administration of intravenous gadolinium contrast in corticomedullary, nephrographic, and urographic phases of renal enhancement.[18]

Gadolinium contrast agents are considered nonnephrotoxic at the dose used for MRI, but administration seems to be associated with nephrogenic systemic fibrosis in patients with severely impaired renal function (<30 mL/min/1.73 m^2).[19–22] The FDA has issued a black box warning for use of gadolinium-based contrast agents in patients with severe renal insufficiency, and the American College of Radiology guidelines recommend refraining from use of gadolinium contrast in such patients unless the risk-benefit assessment for a particular patient clearly favors need for administration.

Assessment of Renal Lesions

As in renal mass evaluation with CT, assessing the presence or absence of enhancement is the most important factor in differentiating benign from malignant renal lesions.[23] This evaluation for enhancement can be performed either qualitatively or as a quantitative measure of change in signal intensity. Subtracting the precontrast acquisition from the contrast-enhanced images facilitates

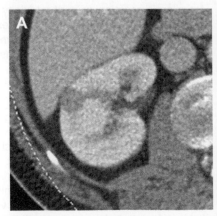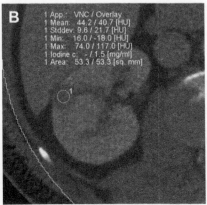

Fig. 3. (*A*) DECT single-phase examination after administration of intravenous contrast demonstrates a mass in the right kidney. (*B*) Enhancement in this lesion is confirmed on iodine overlay image that is generated with 3-material decomposition. This lesion has an iodine concentration greater than 1 mg/mL. Low level of enhancement suggested papillary RCC, confirmed on histopathology after resection.

Table 1 MRI protocol for renal mass evaluation	
Sequence	**Clinical Use**
T1 in and out of phase	Detection of macroscopic and microscopic fat
T2 HASTE	Lesion detection, high water content is bright
Diffusion-weighted sequence, including multi–b value DWI	Lesion cellularity and vascularity (investigational)
Dynamic T1 gradient-echo 3D fat saturation (before and after contrast administration) at following time points:	—
Arterial phase/corticomedullary (no delay)	Vascular anatomy, lesion detection and characterization
Nephrographic (70–90 s)	Best phase for lesion detection and characterization
Urographic/excretory phase (7 minutes)	Relationship of mass to collecting system
Coronal T1 gradient-echo 3D with fat saturation: urogram	Evaluation of collecting system in the coronal plane

Abbreviation: HASTE, half Fourier acquisition single-shot turbo spin-echo.

evaluation for presence of subtle enhancement, particularly in small masses or lesions already bright on precontrast T1 images such as masses containing hemorrhage or hemorrhagic cysts.[24] MRI is also more sensitive than CT for detecting features within cystic lesions, namely, the presence, thickness, and enhancement of septa. When the Bosniak criteria were applied to cystic lesions on MRI, 10% of cases were upstaged.[13] However, clinical significance of this increased contrast resolution on MRI remains unclear.

MRI can detect both macroscopic and microscopic fat, which can help diagnose angiomyolipoma. On T1-weighted out-of-phase images, macroscopic fat demonstrates a black outline called an India ink artifact, which was seen in 100% of angiomyolipomas and 4% nonangiomyolipoma renal lesions in a study by Israel and colleagues.[25]

Microscopic (intravoxel) fat manifests as signal loss on out-of-phase imaging and can increase confidence in the diagnosis of angiomyolipoma with minimal fat (**Fig. 4**). However, clear cell subtype of RCC may also contain intracytoplasmic lipid, and diagnosis of angiomyolipoma should be made with caution in the absence of macroscopic fat.

Staging and surgical planning

In addition to renal mass characterization, both CT and MRI can provide essential information for staging and preoperative planning. Use of ultrasonography for RCC staging is limited by bowel gas and body habitus, which often obscure the renal vein, inferior vena cava, and retroperitoneal lymph nodes. Staging by MDCT and MRI is similarly accurate.

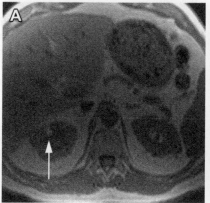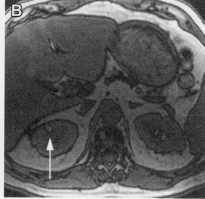

Fig. 4. (*A*) T1 in-phase image demonstrates a right renal lesion that is of high signal intensity. (*B*) On T1 out-of-phase image, there is India ink artifact around its margin compatible with bulk fat, which confirms diagnosis of an angiomyolipoma.

Multiphase acquisition including angiographic phase, multiplanar reformations, and maximum intensity projections are some of the tools available with CT and MRI that supplement anatomic information. CT and magnetic resonance (MR) angiographic acquisition can demonstrate the number of renal arteries, feeding arteries to a mass, and presence of vascular invasion. CT or MR urographic acquisition can delineate tumor proximity to the hilum or collecting system, thus assisting with preoperative planning.

The R.E.N.A.L. Nephrometry Scoring System[26] assigns a numerical score to anatomic descriptors of the tumor, including maximal tumor radius, exophytic versus endophytic nature of the tumor, proximity of the tumor to the collecting system or sinus, location relative to polar lines, and anterior or posterior tumor location. The scoring system has been shown to be a good predictor of surgical outcomes of laparoscopic partial nephrectomy[27] as well as histology and grade of RCCs.[28]

Regarding T staging, evaluation of tumor involvement beyond the renal capsule or Gerota fascia may be better evaluated with MRI than with CT because perirenal fat invasion and fat planes with adjacent structures are better depicted.[29,30] Presence of thrombus in the renal vein and inferior vena cava can also be evaluated and is best seen on contrast-enhanced T1-weighted sequences of MRI as a low-signal filling defect. The negative predictive value of tumor within the renal vein or inferior vena cava is near 100% using MRI.[31] Enhancement of the thrombus suggests intravenous tumor growth rather than bland thrombus. Although the reported sensitivity for detection of venous invasion is 100% in MRI and 79% to 85% in CT,[32] such comparative studies were performed before MDCT became widely available. MRI likely remains better in assessing the cranial extent of venous thrombus because postcontrast CT often does not provide sufficient opacification of the superior-most portion of the IVC to evaluate extension.

Lymphadenopathy is likely equally detected with contrast-enhanced CT and most sequences on MRI, but diagnosis of nodal metastases on both imaging modalities is based on size and is therefore insensitive for metastasis in normal-size lymph nodes.[33]

Evaluation of distant intra-abdominal metastases can be assessed with either CT or MRI, whereas intrathoracic metastatic disease should be evaluated with CT. Positron emission tomography (PET) and PET/CT are also sometimes used for RCC staging, although there is limited sensitivity with the radiotracer fludeoxyglucose F-18 and a negative study does not sufficiently exclude distant metastasis.[34]

ADVANCED MRI TECHNIQUES

Recent advances in functional MRI techniques such as diffusion-weighted imaging (DWI) and perfusion-weighted imaging (PWI) are not yet in widespread clinical use, but potentially offer improved detection and characterization of renal lesions, including prediction of RCC subtype and nuclear grade.

DWI

Brownian motion, or the motion of water molecules, is the basis of image contrast in DWI. Restriction to the mobility of protons in water molecules depends on their environment, which can be qualitatively and quantitatively assessed.[35,36] In highly cellular structures such as tumors, the higher density of cell membranes presumably restricts the diffusion of water protons. The restricted motion is translated into high signal intensity on diffusion-weighted images with a corresponding low apparent diffusion coefficient (ADC), which represents the quantitative measure of diffusion restriction. On the other hand, environments with minimal or no cellularity, such as simply cysts, have higher mobility of water molecules and therefore appear as low signal intensity on diffusion-weighted acquisition with a high corresponding ADC value.

DWI is used in clinical practice along with routine sequences for detection and characterization of renal lesions by visually comparing the differential signal intensity between normal renal parenchyma and lesions. Quantitative ADC values are being examined by several investigators for distinguishing benign and malignant renal lesions, as well as differentiating RCC subtype and grade.

Lesion detection and characterization

Cellular lesions such as RCC demonstrate restricted diffusion on images with higher b value (≥ 400 s/mm^2) compared with normal renal parenchyma (**Fig. 5**).[37–39] Kim and colleagues[40] showed that DWI can differentiate benign and malignant T1 hyperintense renal lesions (without the use of gadolinium contrast), with significantly lower ADC values found in malignant lesions compared with benign lesions (1.75 ± 0.57 vs $2.50 \pm 0.53 \times 10^{-3}$ mm^2/s) using b values of 0, 400, and 800 s/mm^2. The sensitivity and specificity of DWI in accurate characterization of T1 hyperintense renal lesions was 71% and 91%, respectively, and the accuracy in characterizing T1 hyperintense renal lesions was improved when DWI was added

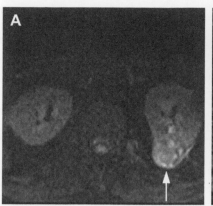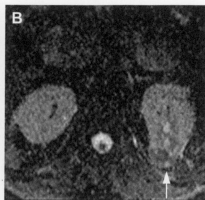

Fig. 5. (A) DWI with b value of 600 s/mm² demonstrates a renal mass at the posterior left kidney, which has areas of high signal intensity. (B) ADC map demonstrates region of low signal intensity (*arrows*), indicating restricted diffusion in a renal neoplasm.

to the routine contrast-enhanced subtraction imaging.

DWI has also been examined for differentiating cystic renal cell neoplasms from benign cysts; lower ADC was found in cystic renal cell neoplasms compared with cysts.[39,41] Taouli and colleagues[39] reported lower mean ADC values in RCC than in benign lesions and also in Bosniak category 3 and 4 lesions than in category 1 simple cysts but did not detect a statistically significant difference in ADC values between Bosniak 2F/benign 3 when compared to Bosniak 4 lesions.

In general, lower ADC values have been shown in the papillary subtype of RCC compared with non papillary subtypes at 1.5 T with b values of 0, 400, and 800 s/mm²,[39] also corroborated at 3.0 T. Wang and colleagues[42] performed DWI with b values of 0 and 500 s/mm² and found that clear cell RCCs showed a significantly higher mean ADC (1.85×10^{-3} mm²/s) than papillary (1.09×10^{-3} mm²/s) and chromophobe (1.31×10^{-3} mm²/s) RCCs. ADC has also been reported to be significantly lower in high nuclear grade (III and IV) than low nuclear grade (I& II) clear cell RCCs.[43] By predicting tumor histology in RCC noninvasively, DWI may potentially help clinical management of RCC.

Assessment of treatment response

Functional imaging techniques such as DWI could potentially aid assessment of response to chemotherapy, given the limitations of size criteria such as RECIST (Response Evaluation Criteria in Solid Tumors) in patients undergoing targeted chemotherapy.[44,45] Changes in ADC have been studied for monitoring treatment response in non-renal primary malignancies,[46,47] and our group and others are currently investigating the potential role

of DWI in assessing response of RCCs to antiangiogenic drugs such as tyrosine kinase inhibitors.[48]

Limitation and future direction

Current limitations in abdominal DWI include a low signal-to-noise ratio, limited spatial resolution, and susceptibility to artifacts such as distortion, ghosting, and blurring that can be somewhat mitigated with technical optimization. The investigation of DWI as a noncontrast-enhanced technique for deriving perfusion information is also under investigation.[49,50] With intravoxel incoherent motion diffusion imaging, tumor perfusion effects may be separated from true diffusion by performing DWI with multiple b values in the low (0–200 s/mm) and high (>200 s/mm) diffusion regimes respectively.[51,52] Thus, perfusion fraction and true diffusion coefficient provide different information about the tumor that may serve as quantitative markers for characterization of malignancies and assessing treatment response.

PWI

Basic principle

As discussed earlier, dynamic contrast-enhanced images are fundamental to renal mass evaluation using MRI and are usually acquired using a 3-dimensional T1-weighted fat-suppressed gradient-echo sequence performed before and after gadolinium contrast administration in the corticomedullary, nephrographic, and urographic phases of enhancement approximately 40 seconds, 100 seconds, and 7 minutes after injection of gadolinium contrast. Although this temporal resolution of 60 seconds or more is sufficient to qualitatively detect enhancement, quantitative parameters of tumor vascularity or perfusion require greater temporal resolution of approximately 5 seconds or less.[35] PWI uses high–temporal resolution imaging for measurement of vascular or perfusional changes in kidneys and renal tumors. After placing regions of interest and generating signal intensity versus time curves, various techniques or models can be used to generate perfusion metrics.

Semiquantitative and quantitative methods are available for analysis of PWI data. The simpler semiquantitative techniques provide parameters such as initial upslope of enhancement, time to peak, and a washout rate but are limited by unclear physiologic or biological correlates for the various parameters. Quantitative analysis entails choosing one of multiple available pharmacokinetic models. Various pharmacokinetic models are being studied by the authors' group and other investigators to identify the best method of quantifying the vascularity and biological behavior of renal tumors.[53]

Lesion characterization
In general, the papillary RCC subtype exhibits low-level homogenous enhancement compared with the clear cell subtype. Papillary RCC can be discriminated from clear cell RCC with high accuracy on the basis of degree of enhancement on corticomedullary phase imaging.[54] In a study using higher temporal resolution of about 30 seconds, a distinct enhancement pattern of an early enhancement peak followed by lower level enhancement was identified in angiomyolipomas.[55]

Assessment of treatment response
Notohamiprodjo and colleagues[56] performed high–temporal resolution PWI and analyzed the data with a 2-compartmental model to generate perfusion and permeability parameters directed toward diagnosing tumor subtype and identifying tumor features such as necrosis and vessel invasion. PWI could potentially aid assessment of response in patients undergoing antiangiogenic drug therapy because changes in tumor size lag behind changes in tumor architecture and perfusion. Several studies have demonstrated qualitative and quantitative changes in various perfusion metrics after antiangiogenic drug therapy.[57,58] Flaherty and colleagues[59] also showed that a high gadolinium exchange constant between serum (blood) and tumor interstitium or transfer coefficient (ktrans) at baseline was associated with better treatment response to sorafenib as well as longer tumor-free survival.

Limitation and future direction
The investigation of PWI for clinical use is evolving but limited by a lack of consensus in the literature regarding pharmacokinetic models and technical imaging parameters to be used in assessment of renal lesions. At present, processing of perfusion data is time intensive and labor intensive, and automated postprocessing tools are under development.

SUMMARY

Imaging is essential to the diagnosis and management of patients with known or suspected RCC. CT and MRI are most often used for renal lesion detection and characterization, in preoperative planning, and for postoperative follow-up evaluation. Advanced imaging techniques in both CT and MRI are being investigated that will further affect management of RCC.

REFERENCES

1. Jayson M, Sanders H. Increased incidence of serendipitously discovered renal cell carcinoma. Urology 1998;51:203–5.
2. Bosniak MA. The small (< = 3.0 cm) renal parenchymal tumor: detection, diagnosis, and controversies. Radiology 1991;179:307–17.
3. Patard JJ, Leray E, Rioux-Leclercq N, et al. Prognostic value of histologic subtypes in renal cell carcinoma: a multicenter experience. J Clin Oncol 2005; 23(12):2763–71.
4. Thompson RH, Kurta JM, Kaag M, et al. Tumor size is associated with malignant potential in renal cell carcinoma. J Urol 2009;181(5):2033–6.
5. Zirinsky K, Auh YH, Rubenstein WA, et al. CT of the hyperdense renal cyst: sonographic correlation. AJR Am J Roentgenol 1984;143(1):151–6.
6. Israel GM, Bosniak MA. How I do it: evaluating renal masses. Radiology 2005;236:441–50.
7. Park BK, Kim B, Kim SH, et al. Assessment of cystic renal masses based on Bosniak classification: comparison of CT and contrast-enhanced US. Eur J Radiol 2007;61(2):310–4.
8. Jamis-Dow CA, Choyke PL, Jennings SB, et al. Small (< or = 3-cm) renal masses: detection with CT versus US and pathologic correlation. Radiology 1996;198:785–8.
9. Yamashita Y, Takahashi M, Watanabe O, et al. Small renal cell carcinoma: pathologic and radiologic correlation. Radiology 1992;184(2):493–8.
10. Ruppert-Kohlmayr AJ, Uggowitzer M, Meissnitzer T, et al. Differentiation of renal clear cell carcinoma and renal papillary carcinoma using quantitative CT enhancement parameters. AJR Am J Roentgenol 2004;183:1387–91.
11. Zhang J, Lefkowitz RA, Ishill NM, et al. Solid renal cortical tumors: differentiation with CT. Radiology 2007;244:494–504.
12. Herts BR, Coll DM, Novick AC, et al. Enhancement characteristics of papillary renal neoplasms

revealed on triphasic helical CT of the kidneys. AJR Am J Roentgenol 2002;178:367–72.

13. Israel GM, Hindman N, Bosniak MA. Evaluation of cystic renal masses: comparison of CT and MR imaging by using the Bosniak classification system. Radiology 2004;231(2):365–71.

14. Fletcher JG, Takahashi N, Hartman R, et al. Dual-energy and dual-source CT: is there a role in the abdomen and pelvis? Radiol Clin North Am 2009;47(1):41–57.

15. Graser A, Becker CR, Staehler M, et al. Single-phase dual-energy CT allows for characterization of renal masses as benign or malignant. Invest Radiol 2010;45(7):399–405.

16. Chandarana H, Megibow AJ, Cohen BA, et al. Iodine quantification with dual-energy CT: phantom study and preliminary experience with renal masses. AJR Am J Roentgenol 2011;196(6):W693–700.

17. Chandarana H, Block TK, Rosenkrantz AB, et al. Free-breathing radial 3D fat-suppressed T1-weighted gradient echo sequence: a viable alternative for contrast-enhanced liver imaging in patients unable to suspend respiration. Invest Radiol 2011; 46(10):648–53.

18. Kang SK, Kim D, Chandarana H. Contemporary imaging of the renal mass. Curr Urol Rep 2011; 112(1):11–7.

19. Sadowski EA, Bennett LK, Chan MR, et al. Nephrogenic systemic fibrosis: risk factors and incidence estimation. Radiology 2007;243(1):148–57.

20. Perez-Rodriguez J, Lai S, Ehst BD, et al. Nephrogenic systemic fibrosis: incidence, associations, and effect of risk factor assessment—report of 33 cases. Radiology 2009;250(2):371–7.

21. Grobner T. Gadolinium—a specific trigger for the development of nephrogenic fibrosing dermopathy and nephrogenic systemic fibrosis? Nephrol Dial Transplant 2006;21(4):1104–8.

22. Kuo P, Kanal E, Abu-Alfa AK, et al. Gadolinium-based MR contrast agents and nephrogenic systemic fibrosis. Radiology 2007;242:647–9.

23. Ho V, Allen S, Hood M, et al. Renal masses: quantitative assessment of enhancement with dynamic MR imaging. Radiology 2002;224:695–700.

24. Hecht EM, Israel GM, Krinsky GA, et al. Renal masses: quantitative analysis of enhancement with signal intensity measurements versus qualitative analysis of enhancement with image subtraction for diagnosing malignancy at MR imaging. Radiology 2004;232:373–8.

25. Israel GM, Hindman N, Hecht E, et al. The use of opposed-phase chemical shift MRI in the diagnosis of renal angiomyolipomas. AJR Am J Roentgenol 2005;184(6):1868–72.

26. Kutikov A, Uzzo RG. The R.E.N.A.L. nephrometry score: a comprehensive standardized system for quantitating renal tumor size, location and depth. J Urol 2009;182(3):844–53.

27. Hayn MH, Schwaab T, Underwood W, et al. RENAL nephrometry score predicts surgical outcomes of laparoscopic partial nephrectomy. BJU Int 2011; 108(6):876–81.

28. Kutikov A, Smaldone MC, Egleston BL, et al. Anatomic features of enhancing renal masses predict malignant and high-grade pathology: a preoperative nomogram using the RENAL nephrometry score. Eur Urol 2011;60:241–8.

29. Narumi Y, Miyazaki T, Hatanaka Y, et al. MR imaging evaluation of renal carcinoma. Abdom Imaging 1997; 22:216–25.

30. Huch boni RA, Debatin JF, Krestin FP. Contrast-enhanced MR imaging of the kidneys and adrenal glands. Magn Reson Imaging Clin N Am 1996;4:101–31.

31. Choyke PL, Walther MM, Wagner JR, et al. Renal cancer: preoperative evaluation with dual phase three-dimensional MR angiography. Radiology 1997; 205(3):767–71.

32. Kallman DA, King BF, Hattery RR, et al. Renal vein and inferior vena cava tumor thrombus in renal cell carcinoma: CT, US, MRI and venacavography. J Comput Assist Tomogr 1992;16(2):240–7.

33. Sohn KM, Lee JM, Lee SY, et al. Comparing MR imaging and CT in the staging of gastric carcinoma [Published erratum appears in AJR Am J Roentgenol 2000;175:556]. AJR Am J Roentgenol 2000; 174:1551–7.

34. Majhail NS, Urbain JL, Albani JM, et al. F-18 fluorodeoxyglucose positron emission tomography in the evaluation of distant metastases from renal cell carcinoma. J Clin Oncol 2003;21:3995–4000.

35. Chandarana H, Taouli B. Diffusion and perfusion imaging of the liver. Eur J Radiol 2010;76(3): 348–58.

36. Thoeny HC, De Keyzer F. Diffusion-weighted MR imaging of native and transplanted kidneys. Radiology 2011;259(1):25–38.

37. Squillaci E, Manenti G, Di Stefano F, et al. Diffusion-weighted MR imaging in the evaluation of renal tumours. J Exp Clin Cancer Res 2004;23: 39–45.

38. Cova M, Squillaci E, Stacul F, et al. Diffusion-weighted MRI in the evaluation of renal lesions: preliminary results. Br J Radiol 2004;77:851–7.

39. Taouli B, Thakur RK, Mannelli L, et al. Renal lesions: characterization with diffusion-weighted imaging versus contrast-enhanced MR imaging. Radiology 2009;251:398–407.

40. Kim S, Jain M, Harris AB, et al. T1 hyperintense renal lesions: characterization with diffusion-weighted MR imaging versus contrast-enhanced MR imaging. Radiology 2009;251:796–807.

41. Sandrasegaran K, Sundaram CP, Ramaswamy R, et al. Usefulness of diffusion-weighted imaging in the evaluation of renal masses. Am J Roent 2010; 194:438–45.

42. Wang H, Cheng L, Zhang X, et al. Renal cell carcinoma: diffusion-weighted MR imaging for subtype differentiation at 3.0 T. Radiology 2010; 257:135–43.

43. Rosenkrantz AB, Niver BE, Fitzgerald EF, et al. Utility of the apparent diffusion coefficient for distinguishing clear cell renal cell carcinoma of low and high nuclear grade. AJR Am J Roentgenol 2010;195: 344–51.

44. Choi H. Response evaluation of gastrointestinal stromal tumors. Oncologist 2008;13(Suppl 2):4–7.

45. Smith AD, Shah SN, Rini BI, et al. Morphology, attenuation, size, and structure (MASS) criteria: assessing response and predicting clinical outcome in metastatic renal cell carcinoma on antiangiogenic targeted therapy. AJR Am J Roentgenol 2010; 194(6):1470–8.

46. Padhani AR, Koh DM. Diffusion MR imaging for monitoring of treatment response. Magn Reson Imaging Clin N Am 2011;19:181–209.

47. Kamel IR, Reyes DK, Liapi E, et al. Functional MR imaging assessment of tumor response after 90Y microsphere treatment in patients with unre hepatocellular carcinoma. J Vasc Interv Radiol 2007;18:49–56.

48. Leary A, Pickering LM, Larkin JMG, et al. Quantitative diffusion-weighted (DW) MR imaging of microcapillary perfusion and tissue diffusivity as biomarkers of response of renal cell carcinoma (RCC) to treatment with sunitinib. Presented at the 2011 American Society of Clinical Oncology Annual Meeting. Chicago (IL). J Clin Oncol 2011;29:Supplement abstract TPS154.

49. Koh DM, Collins DJ, Orton MR. Intravoxel incoherent motion in body diffusion-weighted MRI: reality and challenges. AJR Am J Roentgenol 2011;196(6): 1351–61.

50. Chandarana H, Lee VS, Hecht E, et al. Comparison of biexponential and monoexponential model of diffusion weighted imaging in evaluation of renal lesions: preliminary experience. Invest Radiol 2011; 46(5):285–91.

51. Le Bihan D, Breton E, Lallemand D, et al. Separation of diffusion and perfusion in intravoxel incoherent motion MR imaging. Radiology 1988;168:497–505.

52. Le Bihan D, Breton E, Lallemand D, et al. MR imaging of intravoxel incoherent motions: application to diffusion and perfusion in neurologic disorders. Radiology 1986;161:401–7.

53. Sourbron SP, Buckley DL. On the scope and interpretation of the Tofts models for DCE-MRI. Magn Reson Med 2011;66(3):735–45.

54. Sun MR, Ngo L, Genega EM, et al. Renal cell carcinoma: dynamic contrast-enhanced MR imaging for differentiation of tumor subtypes—correlation with pathologic findings. Radiology 2009;250:793–802.

55. Scialpi M, Di Maggio A, Midiri M, et al. Small renal masses: assessment of lesion characterization and vascularity on dynamic contrast-enhanced MR imaging with fat suppression. AJR Am J Roentgenol 2000;175(3):751–7.

56. Notohamiprodjo M, Sourbron S, Staehler M, et al. Measuring perfusion and permeability in renal cell carcinoma with dynamic contrast-enhanced MRI: a pilot study. J Magn Reson Imaging 2010;31(2):490–501.

57. Hillman GG, Singh-Gupta V, Al-Bashir AK, et al. Dynamic contrast-enhanced magnetic resonance imaging of sunitinib-induced vascular changes to schedule chemotherapy in renal cell carcinoma xenograft tumors. Transl Oncol 2010;3(5):293–306.

58. Galbraith SM, Maxwell RJ, Lodge MA, et al. Combretastatin A4 phosphate has tumor antivascular activity in rat and man as demonstrated by dynamic magnetic resonance imaging. J Clin Oncol 2003;21: 2831–42.

59. Flaherty KT, Rosen MA, Heitjan DF, et al. Pilot study of DCE-MRI to predict progression-free survival with sorafenib therapy in renal cell carcinoma. Cancer Biol Ther 2008;7(4):496–501.

Approach to the Small Renal Mass: to Treat or Not to Treat

Simon P. Kim, MD, MPH, R. Houston Thompson, MD*

KEYWORDS

- Active surveillance • Kidney cancer • Nephrectomy
- Renal cell carcinoma • Small renal masses • Surgery
- Survival • Treatment decisions

In 2010, renal cell carcinoma (RCC) remained the third most commonly diagnosed genitourinary malignancy with an estimated 58,240 incident cases and 8210 cancer-related deaths in the United States.[1] Over the past 2 decades, however, small renal masses (SRMs) have become an increasingly prevalent clinical scenario for urologic surgeons, while management has simultaneously undergone considerable changes in the treatment paradigm. Increasing national use of cross-sectional imaging has been not only presumably responsible for a rising incidence of SRM[2–4] but also implicated in the gradual reduction of clinical stage and primary renal tumor size, such that SRMs (<4 cm) now account for more than a majority of incident cases.[5,6] Contemporary trends of more localized and smaller renal tumors at presentation have nonetheless not translated into significant improvements in survival, which may be because of the highly unpredictable clinical behavior of this lethal malignancy.[3]

The optimal treatment paradigm for SRM has been similarly redefined. Radical nephrectomy (RN) has been the historical treatment of choice for SRM because of its excellent long-term oncologic control for RCC.[7] Yet, emerging evidence suggests that partial nephrectomy (PN) while achieving similar oncologic control, may also confer improved overall survival because of its lower risk of chronic kidney disease and cardiovascular disease than RN.[8–12] Ablative therapy, whether by cryoablation or radiofrequency ablations, has also been shown to provide acceptable oncologic outcomes with intermediate follow-up, although it is widely acknowledged that many of these single-institution series have yet to accrue the sample sizes and follow-up needed to generalize the results to a patient population with SRM.[13] Recent studies suggest that active surveillance of SRM may be another reasonable treatment alternative because of the slow tumor size growth kinetics and low, albeit potentially lethal, risk of progression,[14–16] in particular for those patients with advanced age or multiple comorbidities.[17]

Against this backdrop, SRMs present an increasingly difficult clinical dilemma in determining the ideal treatment while balancing the risks of cancer-related progression and death against the potential benefits and harms from each treatment modality. It would be appealing to assume that the treatment management of SRM would be a one-size-fits-all approach. However, SRMs exhibit marked heterogeneity in clinical behavior for cancer progression. Moreover, treatment decisions to determine whether to proceed with nephrectomy, ablation, or active surveillance remain highly complex and rely on clinical judgments regarding risk of cancer-related progression and death, life expectancy, comorbidities, performance status, and treatment preference. In this context, we describe different treatment options for SRM, in particular active surveillance, and present existing prediction tools that are readily available for clinicians and patients to facilitate informed treatment decisions about the optimal management of SRM. We also review risk-adapted algorithms that take

Funding: None. Disclosures: None.
Department of Urology, Mayo Clinic, 200 First Street Southwest, Rochester, MN 55905, USA
* Corresponding author.
E-mail address: Thompson.Robert@mayo.edu

Urol Clin N Am 39 (2012) 171–179
doi:10.1016/j.ucl.2012.01.003

urologic.theclinics.com

into consideration patient characteristics that may pose risk factors of postoperative complications and exposure to surgical treatment.

TREATMENT ALTERNATIVES AND CLINICAL GUIDELINES FOR SRM

Current clinical guidelines recommend PN as the preferred management of SRM, if technically feasible based on primary tumor size and location.[18–20] Although RN has been the historical gold standard for SRM, several observational studies have demonstrated that PN can provide equivalent long-term cancer-specific survival when compared with RN[21–25] while also reducing the risks of adverse functional renal outcome, cardiovascular events, and all-cause mortality.[8,10–12] For example, Lau and colleagues[25] were among the first to report a matched analysis of patients surgically treated with RN and PN for unilateral RCC at the Mayo Clinic, where the long-term outcomes at 15 years were similar for local (99% vs 95%, $P = .18$) and distant recurrence-free survival (99% vs 95%, $P = .18$) and cancer-specific survival (96% vs 91%, $P = .71$). Likewise, Zini and colleagues[26] used a multi-institutional historical cohort to similarly demonstrate that PN and RN achieved equally low cancer-specific mortality at 5 years (2.1% vs 1.0, P = non-significant).

Although it is generally accepted that both PN and RN confer durable cancer control for T1a and T1b renal tumors, several observational studies have recently indicated that the benefits of PN in comparison with RN may be attributable to the lower risks of chronic kidney disease and, as a result, lower risks of associated cardiovascular disease and all-cause mortality. In 2006, Memorial Sloan-Kettering Cancer Center reported the incidence of new-onset chronic kidney disease from its retrospective cohort of 662 patients with T1a renal tumors who underwent surgical extirpation from 1989 to 2005.[12] In comparison with PN, patients who underwent RN for SRMs were 3.82 times more likely to develop new-onset moderate to severe chronic kidney disease after surgery ($P<.001$). Population-based cohorts from Surveillance, Epidemiology and End Results (SEER)-Medicare also demonstrated the benefits of PN in observing a 26% reduction in adverse renal outcomes (hazard ratio [HR], 0.74; $P<.001$).[10] These observational studies support the findings that PN, with its lower risks of adverse functional renal outcome, also correlated with improved overall survival. Indeed, we previously reported that RN was significantly associated with a 2-fold higher risk of all-cause mortality than PN in a subset of patients younger than 65 years (HR,

2.16; $P = .02$).[8] Another SEER-Medicare population-based study from 1995 to 2002 confirmed these findings in that RN resulted in a higher incidence of cardiovascular disease (HR, 1.4; $P<.05$) and all-cause mortality (HR, 1.38; $P<.01$).[11] The results of these observational studies have served as the basis for the recent changes to the clinical guidelines in recommending PN for SRM. Consequently, PN remains the treatment of choice for those patients having SRMs amenable to resection based on location and tumor size and who are healthy enough to tolerate surgery.[18,27,28]

Ablative therapy with cryoablation or radiofrequency ablation is an alternative treatment option for SRM. Although the indications and outcomes of thermal ablation are discussed in greater detail in another article by Cadeddu and Faddegon in the same issue, it does warrant some discussion here because thermal ablation represents an acceptable treatment alternative for SRM. At present, clinical guidelines recognize cryoablation and radiofrequency ablation as treatment options only in the setting of patients who are poor surgical candidates due to limited life expectancy and multiple comorbidities, among others.[18,19] Although ablative therapy allows for a greater use of minimally invasive percutaneous approaches, the existing evidence is characterized by studies with small sample sizes and insufficient long-term follow-up that limit the ability to fully ascertain whether this form of therapy is as effective for durable cancer control.

A recent systematic review on the treatment of SRMs also underscores that patient populations from single-institution historical cohort studies examining cryoablation include older patients (65.7 vs 61.6 years, $P<.001$) having smaller renal tumors (2.56 vs 3.40 cm, $P<.001$) compared with studies examining nephrectomy. Despite the smaller mean renal tumor size observed in these studies, Kunkle and colleagues[29] also reported a statistically higher risk of local recurrence for cryoablation (relative risk [RR], 7.45; $P<.05$) and radiofrequency ablation (RR, 18.21; $P<.05$) compared with surgery, although the heterogeneity in defining local recurrence as an outcome represents an important obstacle in ascertaining the comparative effectiveness of this treatment modality. We also submit that further observations are needed before determining if one form of ablation (ie, cryoablation) is superior to the other. Another important consideration in evaluating the relative effectiveness of ablative therapy for SRM is that there is a paucity of randomized clinical trials or multi-institutional prospective studies critically assessing the ability of either form of ablative therapy to achieve long-term oncologic control and investigating the potential harms associated with treatment and recurrence.

Active surveillance is another emerging treatment strategy for SRM that has become increasingly relevant for patients and urologists because of the evolving demographics of the US population and the slow growth rate, on average, of SRM. Although the mean age at the time of diagnosis of stage I RCC is currently 60.8 years,[30] the aging of the US population profoundly alters the typical presentation of SRM such that it has been estimated that 69% of patients with newly diagnosed SRM will be 65 years or older by 2030.[31] In this context, there is an ongoing clinical debate about whether patients with limited life expectancy would derive a survival benefit from primary treatment of localized RCC while being exposed to the potential harms from surgery associated with older age and comorbidity.[17,32]

Although a study using SEER-Medicare data suggested more aggressive primary treatment with PN conferring superior survival compared with RN for octogenarians with SRM,[33] a historical cohort study from the Cleveland Clinic found similar 5-year cancer-specific mortality with RN, nephron-sparing intervention, and active surveillance (9.3% vs 4.0% vs 5.8%, $P = .33$).[34] Hollingsworth and colleagues[32] performed a competing risk analysis from SEER-Medicare in which all patients underwent nephrectomy for RCC to elucidate the relationships of age and primary renal tumor size with cancer-specific versus other-cause mortality after nephrectomy was performed. The competing risk analysis revealed that patients with advanced age were far more likely to die from other causes than from RCC after nephrectomy was performed. Taken together, these data suggest advanced age, limited life expectancy, and comorbidity are critically important aspects that should be taken into consideration in identifying the appropriate patients for primary treatment of SRM.[35]

Although it is becoming increasingly acknowledged that poor functional status, extensive comorbidities, and limited life expectancy may compromise the benefits of primary treatment, the relatively slow growth of SRM and low risk of progression to metastatic disease also underscore the potential clinical value of active surveillance in appropriately selected patients. Several observational studies of patients with advanced age or who are medically unfit for surgery have documented that most SRMs have relatively static renal tumor growth on serial radiographic surveillance imaging. For example, the Cleveland Clinic initially described their cohort of patients with advanced age (>75 years) who underwent active surveillance.[14,36] Among the 110 patients placed on active surveillance, the mean growth rate was 0.26 cm per year at a median follow-up of 2 years. Although there

were no cancer-related deaths, only 2 (1.8%) patients subsequently developed distant metastasis.

In a systematic review and meta-analysis of 9 retrospective single-institution studies on the natural history of SRM, the pooled mean growth rate was also 0.28 cm per year, while only 1% of patients progressed to metastatic disease and none of the patients died from RCC.[15] A recent update of the evidence by systematic review further supported the static growth rate of renal tumors and low rates of progression to metastatic disease while on active surveillance.[37] Although previous studies indicate that tumor growth kinetics and initial primary tumor size may not be reliable predictors of progression,[15,36] the findings from this recent meta-analysis contribute to the understanding of the risk of progression by suggesting that the linear and volumetric growth rates are significantly higher in those in whom the condition subsequently progresses.[37] In the only prospective phase 2 clinical trial of active surveillance of 178 older and infirmed patients, the condition progressed locally in 25 patients (14%), as defined by either a growth of 4 cm or more or an annual doubling time, and 2 (1.1%) patients went onto to develop metastatic disease.[38] Approximately a third of patients' renal tumors, however, were observed to have minimal growth on radiographic imaging. Furthermore, in an era of rising health care costs and increased attention to comparative effectiveness research, active surveillance has been put forth as the most cost-effective treatment strategy for SRM compared with immediate nephrectomy.[39]

Although these findings are encouraging in considering active surveillance as an acceptable treatment strategy, these observational studies are subject to selection bias and are underpowered to accurately predict the risk of cancer-related deaths. Furthermore, although a validated protocol on the intensity of computed tomographic surveillance imaging for active surveillance has yet to be established, radiation exposure is becoming an increasingly recognized public health concern for associated secondary malignancies.[40–42] Therefore, active surveillance should not be considered in younger patients who can tolerate nephrectomy, given the lack of high-quality evidence comparing the different treatment options, significant heterogeneity across studies, and the cumulative radiation exposure due to cross-sectional imaging from active surveillance.

PREDICTIVE MODELS FOR SRMs

Treatment decisions for SRM on whether to intervene surgically with PN, RN, and thermal ablation or to use active surveillance require careful deliberation based on the individualized patient and tumor characteristics. For patients to make informed medical decisions on how to treat the SRM, it is essential for physicians to accurately communicate the benefits and risks associated with each treatment modality and active surveillance. In response, prediction models have been developed from surgical cohorts to ascertain the risks of various oncologic end points. These prognostic models can help patients diagnosed with SRM and urologic surgeons to have deliberate discussions on the risks SRM pose for recurrence, metastasis, cancer-specific survival, and overall survival. In addition, using these prediction models in the clinical setting represents one of the first steps in objectively discussing the risks and benefits of each treatment alternative, thereby minimizing subjective assessments that are likely prone to bias and contribute to variations in the use of PN and RN.[43,44]

Several prediction tools and models using only clinical variables available in the preoperative setting have been proposed to facilitate a quantitative assessment in determining the risks of recurrence, progression, and survival (Table 1). For example, Cindolo and colleagues[45] developed a prognostic model for recurrence-free survival using multi-institutional retrospective data from 660 patients who underwent PN or RN for nonmetastatic RCC. From the multivariate model, the candidate variables identified as significantly associated with the primary outcome included clinical presentation (asymptomatic vs symptomatic) and primary tumor size, which were then aggregated into a model for good and poor prognostic groups. Patients in the poor-risk group achieved only a 5-year recurrence-free survival of 68%, whereas the good-risk group had a 5-year recurrence-free survival of 93% ($P<.001$). Likewise, investigators using retrospective institutional data from Johns Hopkins also developed a similar predictive model for recurrence-free survival from 296 patients who underwent open RN for localized RCC.[46] The investigators also similarly dichotomized the risk groups

Table 1
Preoperative prognostic models for SRM

Study	Sample Size	Clinical T Stage	Treatment	Clinical Variables	Outcomes
Cindolo et al,[45] 2003	660	T1-3	PN, RN	Clinical presentation Primary tumor size[a]	Recurrence-free survival
Yaycioglu et al,[46] 2001	296	T1-3	Open RN	Clinical presentation Primary tumor size[a]	Recurrence-free survival
Hutterer et al,[47] 2007	4658	T1-4	PN, RN	Age Symptom presentation[b] Primary tumor size	Presence of nodal metastasis at the time of nephrectomy
Raj et al,[48] 2008	2517	NA[c]	PN, RN	Gender Mode of presentation[b] Lymphadenopathy or necrosis present on imaging Primary tumor size	12-y probability of metastasis-free survival
Karakiewicz et al,[49] 2009	2474	T1-3 M0-1	PN, RN	Age Gender Symptom classification[b] Tumor size Primary T stage Presence of metastasis	Cancer-specific mortality
Hollingsworth et al,[32] 2007	26,618	T1-2	PN, RN	Age Primary tumor size	Cancer-related and other-cause mortality
Kutikov et al,[50] 2010		T1-2	PN, RN	Age Gender Race Primary tumor size	Kidney cancer–related, other cancer–related, and noncancer–related mortality

[a] Asymptomatic versus symptomatic.
[b] Asymptomatic versus systemic.
[c] The cohort included localized SRMs without any presence of regional or metastatic disease.

into low and high risk by a recurrence risk score. Limitations of both models include the lack of an external validation cohort and a modest predictive accuracy (65%–67%) of recurrence-free survival.

Hutterer and colleagues[47] also contributed to prognostic models by advancing a nomogram to predict the presence of nodal metastasis using retrospective data from 4658 patients who underwent PN or RN with lymphadenectomy from 12 European institutions. The conceptual framework behind the development of this nomogram was to more accurately identify which patients may benefit from a lymphadenectomy or adjuvant therapy. In this study, the investigators also performed development and validation analyses, yielding relatively strong predictive accuracy (78%). In addition, Raj and colleagues[48] also constructed and externally validated a nomogram to predict the development of metastatic disease at 12 years after PN or RN from Memorial Sloan-Kettering and Mayo Clinic. Clinical variables selected for inclusion in the nomogram were gender, mode of presentation, presence of lymphadenopathy or necrosis on preoperative imaging, and primary tumor size. Overall, the nomogram predicting 12-year metastatic-free survival using the selected pretreatment variables exhibited relative strong accuracy in the development (82%) and external validation (76%) cohorts. In another nomogram, Karakiewicz and colleagues[49] developed and externally validated a nomogram to predict cancer-specific mortality using a large retrospective multi-institutional cohort of patients who underwent nephrectomy for localized and metastatic RCC. Given the larger sample size in the study, it was possible to incorporate more clinical variables with stronger predictive accuracy for cancer-specific mortality in this pretreatment nomogram (84%–88%).

A central limitation of the aforementioned models, which facilitate informed treatment decision for patients diagnosed with SRM, is that they focus solely on prognosticating oncologic outcome among patients undergoing nephrectomy. To address this limitation, competing risk analysis has been brought forth as one method to create a standardized comparative analysis of cancer-related mortality versus other-cause mortality to help identify those patients with SRM who are unlikely to derive any improved cancer-specific survival from nephrectomy, because many of these individuals are far more likely to die from other causes. The inference from competing risk analysis is that some patients with limited life expectancy will die from other causes before experiencing any treatment benefit from nephrectomy with improved cancer-specific survival. Using SEER, Hollingsworth and colleagues[32] performed a competing

risks analysis in a population-based cohort to report that the benefits of PN or RN were attenuated by age and tumor size, such that approximately a third of patients aged 70 years or more would die from other causes after surgery. Moreover, although the 5-year competing risk for cancer-specific mortality increased with age, the efficacy of surgical extirpation was significantly mitigated by tumor size, where patients aged 80 years or more with renal tumors smaller than 2 cm were estimated to have a 5-year cancer-related mortality rate at 9.6% versus 54.8% of those who would die due to other causes. Likewise, Kutikov and colleagues[50] also performed a competing risk analysis of kidney cancer–related, other cancer–related, and noncancer-related causes of death using SEER data from 1998 to 2003 in surgically treated patients. In this study, the investigators identified age, race, sex, and primary tumor size as clinically significant variables to construct individual nomograms for kidney cancer–related, other cancer–related, and noncancer-related mortality. Overall, age was most predictive of nonkidney cancer–related mortality, although increasing tumor size was inversely associated with death from kidney cancer. In this competing risk nomogram, a 75-year-old man with a 4-cm renal tumor would have a 5-year mortality estimated at 5% for RCC, 5% for other cancers, and 14% for all other causes. Both the aforementioned competing risk analyses only included patients who were treated with nephrectomy, which thereby mitigated the competing risk of cancer-related death.

Although these models provide some degree of quantitative information detailing the risks of recurrence, metastasis, and survival for patients undergoing nephrectomy for RCC, it is also important to acknowledge the several limitations these tools have in facilitating high-quality treatment decisions in the management of SRM. The existing studies are subject to selection bias, in the sense that all the models are based on surgical cohorts of patients who underwent nephrectomy. At present, these models have not incorporated the true relative benefit of treatment, whether by nephrectomy or thermal ablation, because none of the studies include patients who were not treated and received active surveillance. For patients to make a fully informed decision about the effectiveness of primary therapy, the patient and the surgeon must carefully deliberate the risks of progression and cancer-related death if the SRMs were left untreated. In a recent decision-analytic study using a Markov model to compare the different primary treatment options on incremental life expectancy gain, PN offered an incremental benefit of 4.8 months compared with RN, 7.7 months compared with thermal ablation, and 9.5 months compared with active surveillance.[51] However, among patients older than 74 years at the time of diagnosis, the decision analysis suggested that active surveillance was the preferred treatment.

There is also marked differences and heterogeneity in the patient characteristics (age), primary tumor size, and duration of follow-up in the existing evidence for PN, RN, thermal ablation, and active surveillance such that it is difficult to accurately compare each primary therapy for oncologic outcomes, complications, and harm. It is also necessary to critically evaluate the level of evidence to which we use to guide the development of clinical guidelines and incorporate into clinical practice to better inform our patients of the different treatment options and outcomes for SRM. To date, the existing evidence relies mostly on historical observational studies using institutional or population-based data. At present, only one randomized controlled trial was performed for SRM, which recently suggested that the PN and RN have similar outcomes for cancer-specific survival and overall survival, although the study was underpowered with significant crossover of treatments after randomization.[28,52]

Nonetheless, the current prediction models provide one mechanism to facilitate identifying which patients are most likely to benefit from PN or RN, while taking into account other clinical variables that may attenuate treatment effect or expose high-risk patients to potentially life-threatening complications. In the current American Urological Association guidelines, PN is the preferred treatment for healthy patients diagnosed with an SRM (<4 cm), although active surveillance and thermal ablation can also be offered as treatment alternatives for those who have major comorbidites or high surgical risk (although these patient-level factors are not clearly defined).[18] In a recent review, Gill and colleagues[53] also put forth a risk-adapted algorithm that dichotomized patients into good and poor surgical candidates according to age, major comorbidities, life expectancy, and surgical risk. For patients who were good surgical candidates (age <70 years, no major comorbidities, and good life expectancy and surgical risk), nephrectomy was the preferred treatment, with PN as the treatment of choice if technically feasible. It is unclear whether thermal ablation is an acceptable treatment in patients with a longer life expectancy, given the concerns of local recurrence and radiation exposure from surveillance imaging. At present, thermal ablation for healthy patients diagnosed with an SRM may be considered a second-line treatment option. For poor surgical candidates (age ≥70 years, comorbidities, limited life expectancy, compromised renal function, and poor surgical risk), the preferred primary treatment strategy would involve active surveillance or thermal ablation with possible needle biopsy. Although this algorithm may be potentially useful in the clinical setting to serve as the basis for initiating a discussion on all the important facets of the treatment decision, it is based on expert opinion rather than high-level evidence. Nonetheless, we present a risk-adapted approach for an incidental SRM that takes into consideration

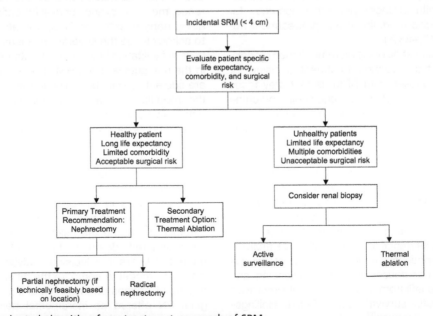

Fig. 1. Risk-adapted algorithm for a treatment approach of SRM.

possible clinical factors, such as life expectancy and comorbidities, that should be discussed and reviewed with patients to make an informed treatment decision (**Fig. 1**).

SUMMARY

Accurately conveying the benefits and risks of treatment interventions to patients diagnosed with SRM is essential to appropriately identify which patients will a achieve better oncologic outcome and confer a survival advantage from primary therapy, while avoiding treatment for those patients who are unlikely to receive a survival benefit or may be unnecessarily exposed to surgical morbidity and mortality. The treatment decision should rely on objective assessments regarding the characteristics of the SRM and risk of progression balanced against a patient's life expectancy, comorbidities, performance status, and treatment preference. For patients who are relatively young with limited comorbidites and acceptable surgical risk, nephrectomy remains the treatment of choice and, if technically feasible, PN is the preferred treatment. However, patients who have limited life expectancy, major comorbidities, or poor surgical risk may be better served by active surveillance or thermal ablation. Existing prediction tools that incorporate key clinical variables, such as age, life expectancy, and primary tumor size, among others, may facilitate an informed decision regarding the best management of SRM by more appropriately selecting treatment individualized to the characteristics of the SRM and a patient's clinical characteristics. Further research is needed in developing validated prediction tools for the primary treatment of SRM by ascertaining the relative effectiveness of nephrectomy, thermal ablation, and active surveillance. On developing these prognostic tools, emphasis should be placed on making them readily available for widespread dissemination into routine clinical practice. Although active surveillance and thermal ablation have been preliminarily promising as acceptable treatment options for SRM, more rigorous evaluation is needed by either randomized trials or prospective multi-institutional studies before these treatment modalities are conclusively considered safe and effective.

REFERENCES

1. Jemal A, Siegel R, Xu J, et al. Cancer statistics, 2010. CA Cancer J Clin 2010;60(5):277–300.
2. Bhargavan M, Sunshine JH. Utilization of radiology services in the United States: levels and trends in modalities, regions, and populations. Radiology 2005;234(3):824–32.
3. Hollingsworth JM, Miller DC, Daignault S, et al. Rising incidence of small renal masses: a need to reassess treatment effect. J Natl Cancer Inst 2006; 98(18):1331–4.
4. Chow WH, Devesa SS, Warren JL, et al. Rising incidence of renal cell cancer in the United States. JAMA 1999;281(17):1628–31.
5. Pantuck AJ, Zisman A, Belldegrun AS. The changing natural history of renal cell carcinoma. J Urol 2001;166(5):1611–23.
6. Kane CJ, Mallin K, Ritchey J, et al. Renal cell cancer stage migration: analysis of the National Cancer Data Base. Cancer 2008;113(1):78–83.
7. Robson CJ, Churchill BM, Anderson W. The results of radical nephrectomy for renal cell carcinoma. J Urol 1969;101(3):297–301.
8. Thompson RH, Boorjian SA, Lohse CM, et al. Radical nephrectomy for pT1a renal masses may be associated with decreased overall survival compared with partial nephrectomy. J Urol 2008;179(2): 468–71 [discussion: 472–3].
9. Thompson RH, Siddiqui S, Lohse CM, et al. Partial versus radical nephrectomy for 4 to 7 cm renal cortical tumors. J Urol 2009;182(6):2601–6.
10. Miller DC, Schonlau M, Litwin MS, et al. Renal and cardiovascular morbidity after partial or radical nephrectomy. Cancer 2008;112(3):511–20.
11. Huang WC, Elkin EB, Levey AS, et al. Partial nephrectomy versus radical nephrectomy in patients with small renal tumors—is there a difference in mortality and cardiovascular outcomes? J Urol 2009;181(1): 55–61 [discussion: 61–2].
12. Huang WC, Levey AS, Serio AM, et al. Chronic kidney disease after nephrectomy in patients with renal cortical tumours: a retrospective cohort study. Lancet Oncol 2006;7(9):735–40.
13. Van Poppel H, Becker F, Cadeddu JA, et al. Treatment of localised renal cell carcinoma. Eur Urol 2011;60(4):662–72.
14. Abouassaly R, Lane BR, Novick AC. Active surveillance of renal masses in elderly patients. J Urol 2008;180(2):505–8 [discussion: 508–9].
15. Chawla SN, Crispen PL, Hanlon AL, et al. The natural history of observed enhancing renal masses: meta-analysis and review of the world literature. J Urol 2006;175(2):425–31.
16. Crispen PL, Viterbo R, Fox EB, et al. Delayed intervention of sporadic renal masses undergoing active surveillance. Cancer 2008;112(5):1051–7.
17. Abouassaly R, Alibahi SM, Tomilson GA, et al. The effect of age on the morbidity of kidney surgery. J Urol 2011;186(3):811–6.
18. Campbell SC, Novick AC, Belldegrun A, et al. Guideline for management of the clinical T1 renal mass. J Urol 2009;182(4):1271–9.

19. Motzer RJ, Agarwal N, Beard C, et al. NCCN clinical practice guidelines in oncology: kidney cancer. 2011. Available at: http://www.nccn.org/professionals/physician_gls/pdf/kidney.pdf. Accessed December 1, 2011.

20. Ljungberg B, Cowan NC, Hanbury DC, et al. EAU guidelines on renal cell carcinoma: the 2010 update. Eur Urol 2010;58(3):398–406.

21. Becker F, Siemer S, Hack M, et al. Excellent long-term cancer control with elective nephron-sparing surgery for selected renal cell carcinomas measuring more than 4 cm. Eur Urol 2006;49(6):1058–63 [discussion: 1063–4].

22. Becker F, Siemer S, Humke U, et al. Elective nephron sparing surgery should become standard treatment for small unilateral renal cell carcinoma: long-term survival data of 216 patients. Eur Urol 2006;49(2):308–13.

23. Leibovich BC, Blute ML, Cheville JC, et al. Nephron sparing surgery for appropriately selected renal cell carcinoma between 4 and 7 cm results in outcome similar to radical nephrectomy. J Urol 2004;171(3): 1066–70.

24. Kim SP, Weight CJ, Leibovich BC, et al. Outcomes and clinicopathologic variables associated with late recurrence after nephrectomy for localized renal cell carcinoma. Urology 2011;78(5):1101–6.

25. Lau WK, Blute ML, Weaver AL, et al. Matched comparison of radical nephrectomy vs nephron-sparing surgery in patients with unilateral renal cell carcinoma and a normal contralateral kidney. Mayo Clin Proc 2000;75(12):1236–42.

26. Zini L, Patard JJ, Capitanio U, et al. Cancer-specific and non-cancer-related mortality rates in European patients with T1a and T1b renal cell carcinoma. BJU Int 2009;103(7):894–8.

27. Joudi FN, Allareddy V, Kane CJ, et al. Analysis of complications following partial and total nephrectomy for renal cancer in a population based sample. J Urol 2007;177(5):1709–14.

28. Van Poppel H, Da Pozzo L, Albrecht W, et al. A prospective randomized EORTC intergroup phase 3 study comparing the complications of elective nephron-sparing surgery and radical nephrectomy for low-stage renal cell carcinoma. Eur Urol 2007; 51(6):1606–15.

29. Kunkle DA, Egleston BL, Uzzo RG. Excise, ablate or observe: the small renal mass dilemma—a meta-analysis and review. J Urol 2008;179(4):1227–33 [discussion: 1233–4].

30. Cooperberg MR, Mallin K, Kane CJ, et al. Treatment trends for stage I renal cell carcinoma. J Urol 2011; 186(2):394–9.

31. Smith BD, Smith GL, Hurria A, et al. Future of cancer incidence in the United States: burdens upon an aging, changing nation. J Clin Oncol 2009;27(17): 2758–65.

32. Hollingsworth JM, Miller DC, Daignault S, et al. Five-year survival after surgical treatment for kidney cancer: a population-based competing risk analysis. Cancer 2007;109(9):1763–8.

33. Hellenthal NJ, Mansour AM, Hayn MH, et al. Renal cell carcinoma in octogenarians: nephron sparing surgery should remain the standard of care. J Urol 2011;185(2):415–20.

34. Lane BR, Abouassaly R, Gao T, et al. Active treatment of localized renal tumors may not impact overall survival in patients aged 75 years or older. Cancer 2010;116(13):3119–26.

35. Lund L, Jacobsen J, Norgaard M, et al. The prognostic impact of comorbidities on renal cancer, 1995 to 2006: a Danish population based study. J Urol 2009;182(1):35–40 [discussion: 40].

36. Abou Youssif T, Kassouf W, Steinberg J, et al. Active surveillance for selected patients with renal masses: updated results with long-term follow-up. Cancer 2007;110(5):1010–4.

37. Smaldone MC, Kutikov A, Egleston BL, et al. Small renal masses progressing to metastases under active surveillance: a systematic review and pooled analysis. Cancer 2011. DOI:10.1002/cncr.26369. [Epub ahead of print].

38. Jewett MA, Mattar K, Basiuk J, et al. Active surveillance of small renal masses: progression patterns of early stage kidney cancer. Eur Urol 2011;60(1):39–44.

39. Heilbrun ME, Yu J, Smith KJ, et al. The cost-effectiveness of immediate treatment, percutaneous biopsy and active surveillance for the diagnosis of the small solid renal mass: evidence from a Markov model. J Urol 2012;187(1):39–43. [Epub 2011 Nov 16].

40. Smith-Bindman R, Lipson J, Marcus R, et al. Radiation dose associated with common computed tomography examinations and the associated lifetime attributable risk of cancer. Arch Intern Med 2009;169(22):2078–86.

41. Brenner DJ, Hall EJ. Computed tomography—an increasing source of radiation exposure. N Engl J Med 2007;357(22):2277–84.

42. Brenner D, Elliston C, Hall E, et al. Estimated risks of radiation-induced fatal cancer from pediatric CT. AJR Am J Roentgenol 2001;176(2):289–96.

43. Dulabon LM, Lowrance WT, Russo P, et al. Trends in renal tumor surgery delivery within the United States. Cancer 2010;116(10):2316–21.

44. Kim SP, Shah ND, Weight CJ, et al. Contemporary trends in nephrectomy for renal cell carcinoma in the United States: results from a population based cohort. J Urol 2011;186(5):1779–85.

45. Cindolo L, de la Taille A, Messina G, et al. A preoperative clinical prognostic model for non-metastatic renal cell carcinoma. BJU Int 2003;92(9):901–5.

46. Yaycioglu O, Roberts WW, Chan T, et al. Prognostic assessment of nonmetastatic renal cell carcinoma: a clinically based model. Urology 2001;58(2):141–5.

47. Hutterer GC, Patard JJ, Perrotte P, et al. Patients with renal cell carcinoma nodal metastases can be accurately identified: external validation of a new nomogram. Int J Cancer 2007;121(11):2556–61.

48. Raj GV, Thompson RH, Leibovich BC, et al. Preoperative nomogram predicting 12-year probability of metastatic renal cancer. J Urol 2008;179(6):2146–51 [discussion: 2151].

49. Karakiewicz PI, Suardi N, Capitanio U, et al. A preoperative prognostic model for patients treated with nephrectomy for renal cell carcinoma. Eur Urol 2009;55(2):287–95.

50. Kutikov A, Egleston BL, Wong YN, et al. Evaluating overall survival and competing risks of death in patients with localized renal cell carcinoma using a comprehensive nomogram. J Clin Oncol 2010; 28(2):311–7.

51. Abouassaly R, Yang S, Finelli A, et al. What is the best treatment strategy for incidentally detected small renal masses? A decision analysis. BJU Int 2011;108(8):E223–31.

52. Van Poppel H, Da Pozzo L, Albrecht W, et al. A prospective, randomised EORTC intergroup phase 3 study comparing the oncologic outcome of elective nephron-sparing surgery and radical nephrectomy for low-stage renal cell carcinoma. Eur Urol 2011;59(4):543–52.

53. Gill IS, Aron M, Gervais DA, et al. Clinical practice. Small renal mass. N Engl J Med 2010;362(7): 624–34.

Does Renal Mass Ablation Provide Adequate Long-term Oncologic Control?

Stephen Faddegon, MD, Jeffrey A. Cadeddu, MD*

KEYWORDS

- Renal neoplasm • Radiofrequency ablation • Cryoablation
- Small renal mass

Although radiofrequency ablation (RFA) and cryotherapy were first described more than 10 years ago,[1,2] large patient series are only now maturing with long-term follow-up. Because these techniques are still new, evidence and expert opinion are constantly evolving. For instance, a Cochrane Review comparing RFA with cryoablation was initially published in 2009 and withdrawn shortly thereafter, in May 2011, possibly because the evidence had already become outdated. There are no randomized studies comparing renal ablation (RA) with surgery or active surveillance. A few meta-analyses have been published in the last 5 years, most comparing surgery with RA and a few comparing RFA with cryoablation. Most of the evidence exists in the form of individual case series and cohort studies. With these limited and biased sources, this article focuses on the ablation series with the longest reported follow-up, and discusses some of the pitfalls in interpreting the literature. Although several different ablation modalities have been described (**Box 1**), only RFA and cryoablation are widely used and have sufficient data to comment on oncologic efficacy. They are the focus of this article.

THE RATIONALE FOR RA

RA has garnered increasing interest with the increase in detection of small renal masses (SRMs).[3] Although 20% to 25% of SRMs prove to be benign, even the malignant neoplasms tend to be less aggressive and of lower grade than their larger counterparts.[4] Although younger patients have traditionally been counseled to undergo surgical treatment of these masses, active surveillance alone is associated with low rates of metastasis. RA might be considered to be on a continuum between surgical excision and surveillance, offering the opportunity for treatment and minimizing patient morbidity.

RA has several advantages compared with partial nephrectomy (PN), including decreased morbidity and better preservation of renal function. Percutaneous ablation is performed as an outpatient procedure with minimal recovery time.[5] In comparative studies with PN, laparoscopic cryoablation (LCA) had reduced blood loss and complication rates,[6] and RFA had better preservation of renal function.[7]

INDICATIONS FOR RA

RA has traditionally been reserved for patients who are poor candidates for surgery or in whom renal preservation is paramount (**Box 2**). However, with some reports of oncologic efficacy approaching that of PN, some centers are now considering RA as a first-line option for young and healthy patients with small tumors.[3,8,9] Although the American Urological Association (AUA) "Guideline for Management of the Clinical Stage 1 Renal Mass"

Statement of disclosures and conflicts of interest: All authors have nothing to disclose.
Department of Urology, University of Texas Southwestern Medical Center, 5323 Harry Hines Boulevard, J8.106, Dallas, TX 75390, USA
* Corresponding author.
E-mail address: Jeffrey.Cadeddu@UTsouthwestern.edu

Box 1
Ablation modalities

- RFA
- Cryotherapy
- High-intensity focused ultrasound (HIFU)
- Laser interstitial thermotherapy (LITT)
- Microwave thermoablation (MWT)
- Pulsed cavitational ultrasound (PCU)
- Chemoablation
- Radiosurgery

---

lists RA as an option for T1b tumors in patients with comorbidities,[10] the authors and others[8] think that tumors larger than 4 cm should seldom be treated with RA, even in patients with comorbidities, because of significantly higher rates of treatment failure and recurrence. The focus of this article is oncologic efficacy for SRMs (ie, cT1a), which is the target population of most series in the literature.

WHAT CONSTITUTES LONG-TERM ONCOLOGIC SUCCESS?

In general, long-term oncologic success requires 5-year and 10-year survival data that encompass

---

Box 2
Indications and contraindications for renal mass ablation

- Well-accepted indications: T1a tumor and
  - Elderly patients
  - Comorbidities/not surgical candidates
  - Renal impairment
  - Multiple bilateral renal masses
- Controversial indications:
  - Small tumors in young/healthy patients
  - Cytoreduction
  - T1b tumors
- Contraindications:
  - Relative
    - Central or hilar tumors
    - Acute illness or infection
    - Unstable cardiovascular status
    - Poor life expectancy
  - Absolute
    - Uncorrected coagulopathy

---

the period in which most recurrences present. However, there are few series with a minimum 5 years of follow-up: 2 LCA series,[11,12] and 1 RFA series from our institution that has been submitted for publication. The focus of this review is therefore series with the longest available follow-up, although many of these series would be strictly defined as having intermediate follow-up.

Oncologic success encompasses local recurrence rates as well as the incidence of metastasis, cancer-specific deaths, and overall survival. Local recurrence is widely defined as new nodular enhancement of the treated lesion on imaging. Although lesions treated by cryoablation generally shrink, RFA-treated lesions may remain stable in size.[13] Furthermore, empiric renal biopsy immediately following RA is generally not performed. In particular, biopsy soon after RFA may have a high false-positive rate. Several studies have suggested residual tumor early after RFA treatment (either on biopsy or PN specimens), whereas others using vitality stains or delayed biopsy more than 12 months after treatment showed that cross-sectional imaging reliably predicted RFA efficacy.[9,14,15] Because early biopsy results and variable changes in lesion size seen after cryoablation do not accurately reflect RA efficacy, treatment success is defined by contrast-enhanced imaging.

To further complicate this definition, there is inconsistency in how local recurrence rates are reported in the literature. The AUA guidelines and several ablation series define local recurrence as any radiographic enhancement at any time after initial therapy. Other series do not consider incomplete treatment as a local recurrence. Instead, these patients are defined as treatment failures that are immediately reablated. In the evaluation of long-term oncologic success, the rate of initial ablation failure requiring retreatment is less relevant than the rate of de novo detection after negative postablation imaging. Although retreatment is inconvenient, costly, and may increase overall complication rate, the necessity to reablate has not be shown to predispose to delayed recurrence, metastasis, or decreased cancer-specific survival, which are the most important oncologic outcomes for the patient.

MAKING SENSE OF DIFFERING EFFICACY RATES BETWEEN RA SERIES

Reports of oncologic efficacy of RA may vary widely between series. For example, a cohort study by Turna and collegeaues[16] found disease-free survival rates for laparoscopic partial nephrectomy (LPN), cryoablation, and RFA to be 100%, 69.6%, and 33.2% respectively (P<.001). In contrast, another cohort study by Takaki and collegeaues[17] found 5-year disease-free survival rates of 95% and 98% for RFA and radical nephrectomy respectively. How can there be such wide variability in reported success between series? **Box 3** outlines several potential explanations.

RA studies can be riddled with biases because there are no randomized studies to control for confounding variables. Different series contain different tumor locations and mean tumor sizes, both of which are known predictors of ablation success.[18,19] In one study, tumors greater than 3.7 cm were associated with higher rates of incomplete ablation and tumor recurrence.[20] Centrally located tumors also have lower efficacy, possibly related to their proximity to vessels that may act as heat sinks.[10,21] In a cohort study comparing RFA with cryoablation, Hegarty and colleagues[22] reported higher rates of incomplete ablation following RFA, although the RFA-treated tumors were more likely to be central (37% vs 6% for cryoablation). In addition, some series correctly report oncologic outcomes only for tumors with a positive pretreatment biopsy, whereas other series include all outcomes, of which 20% to 25% may have benign masses.[4] One meta-analysis showed that pretreatment biopsies were performed in only 82.3% and 62.2% of lesions undergoing cryoablation and RFA respectively.[23]

Oncologic success can also be affected by ablation technique. A lack of standardization makes it difficult to compare series with different ablative technologies, surgical approaches, and levels of experience. For percutaneous RA, many practitioners, including ourselves, also think the type of patient anesthesia affects success. Compared with intravenous sedation, general anesthesia may allow better targeting by controlling respiratory movement.[3,24]

The procedural approach (laparoscopic vs percutaneous) may affect oncologic success for several reasons. Laparoscopic-assisted RA is performed exclusively by surgeons, whereas the percutaneous approach is performed by both surgeons and interventionalists.[25] It has been postulated that surgeons may be more aggressive in treating renal cancer,[26] translating to better outcomes for neoplasms treated by a laparoscopic-assisted approach. A meta-analysis of RFA and cryoablation that compared laparoscopic and percutaneous approaches showed higher rates of primary treatment success in the laparoscopic versus percutaneous group (94% vs 87% respectively, $P<.05$). RFA is more often performed percutaneously, whereas most cryoablation series describe a laparoscopic approach.[8] This discrepancy may explain why one meta-analysis found higher rates of incomplete ablation for RFA compared with cryoablation.[23]

Box 3
Variations between RA series that contribute to conflicting reports of oncologic efficacy

- Selection bias
  - Variable pretreatment renal biopsy practices
  - Variable tumor location or mean tumor size
- Variable reporting of treatment failure:
  - Controversial distinction between local recurrence versus treatment failure
  - Definition of local recurrence (ie, whether based on imaging, biopsy, and so forth)
- Technical variations:
  - Radiologist versus urologist performed
  - Approach (laparoscopic vs percutaneous vs open)
  - Center experience
  - Tumor targeting: computed tomography versus ultrasound guidance
  - Type of sedation: general versus intravenous sedation
  - Variations in ablation technique:
    - Number of electrodes
    - The number of ablation cycles/length of ablation cycle

LONG-TERM OUTCOMES OF RFA

For many years there were only 2 small RFA series with long-term follow-up. These series date back to the early experience with RFA when only patients with significant comorbidities were considered candidates. One-third of the patients in both series died of other causes before long-term oncologic follow-up could mature. In one of these series, Levinson and colleagues[27] reported on 18 patients with pathologically proven renal cell carcinoma (RCC) and a mean follow-up of 57.4 months (range 41–80 months). Recurrence-free survival was suboptimal at 80%, although the actuarial cancer-specific and metastasis-free survival were both 100%. McDougal and colleagues[28] reported a 91% recurrence-free survival in 16 patients with histologically confirmed RCC less than 5 cm in diameter and a minimum of

4 years follow-up. Again, there were no cases of metastasis or cancer-specific deaths.

More recently, Tracy and colleagues[29] reported their RFA series of 243 SRMs with mean tumor size of 2.4 cm and mean follow-up of 27 months (range 1.5–90 months). Considering only the 179 tumors with histologically confirmed RCC, actuarial 5-year survival analysis revealed recurrence-free, metastasis-free, and cancer-specific survival rates of 90%, 95%, and 99% respectively. Similarly, Ferakis and colleagues[30] reported on 31 patients with 39 tumors undergoing percutaneous RFA. Initial ablation success rate was 90% but, when reablation was allowed, the 3-year and actuarial 5-year recurrence-free survival rates were 92% and 89% after a mean follow-up of 61 months (range 36–84 months). These survival estimates likely overestimate the true RCC treatment success because no tumors were biopsied. Furthermore, although the investigators state that the results are comparable with nephron-sparing surgery, recurrence-free rates for PN are widely thought to be greater than 95%.[10] Coupled with the wide confidence intervals that are common in RA series limited by small numbers, comments regarding equivalency to partial nephrectomy cannot be made with any certainty.

Zagoria and colleagues[20] reported their series of 48 histologically proven RCC in 41 patients with median follow-up of 56 months. There were 3 treatment failures (7%), 2 delayed local recurrences (4%), and 3 patients who developed metastasis (7%), 1 of whom died a cancer-related death. There were no recurrences in patients with neoplasms less than 4 cm in diameter. The investigators defined local recurrence as any radiologic enhancement after 1 ablation, yielding local recurrence-free and disease-free survival rates of 88% and 83%.[20]

In summary, the rate of local recurrence after RFA depends partially on definition. If primary treatment failures are considered a local recurrence (ie, patients requiring immediate reablation for persisting enhancement), local recurrence-free survival rates range from 33.2% to 88%.[16,20] When only the cases of recurrence following satisfactory ablation are considered, local recurrence-free survival generally increases to 90% to 95%.[29,30] Metastasis-free and cancer-specific survival are high, consistently greater than 90% across series. **Table 1** summarizes RFA series with intermediate-term and long-term follow-up.

LONG-TERM OUTCOMES OF CRYOTHERAPY

Cryoablation is the most used and studied of all ablative modalities, with a few studies reporting follow-up of 5 years. Guazzoni and colleagues[12] reported favorable oncologic outcomes following LCA in a subgroup analysis of 44 patients with histologically confirmed RCC and a minimum follow-up of 5 years. After a mean follow-up of 61.3 ($\pm$13.8) months, there was 1 local recurrence. There were no cases of cancer-related death and overall survival was 93.2%. Similarly, Weld and colleagues[31] reported 100% 3-year cancer-specific survival, no cases of metastasis, and only 1 case of local recurrence in 31 patients treated by LCA after a mean follow-up of 45.7 months. However, only 22 patients in their series had a biopsy confirming malignancy. Similarly, Davol and colleagues[32] reported their series of 48 patients with a median follow-up of 64 months (range, 36–110 months). In the subgroup with histologically proven RCC, disease-free survival was 84.3% after a single LCA procedure and the cancer-specific survival rate was 100%.

In comparison, a highly experienced center with the longest available follow-up to date for LCA had more sobering results. Considering only the 55 patients with pathologically confirmed RCC who had a minimum 60 months and median 93 month follow-up, 5-year disease-free, cancer-specific, and overall survival rates were 81%, 92%, and 84% respectively.[11]

In summary, cryoablation results in long-term disease-free survival rates of 80% or higher and cancer-specific survival greater than 90% in most series. **Table 2** summarizes cryoablation series with intermediate-term and long-term follow-up.

ARE RFA AND CRYOTHERAPY EQUIVALENT?

RFA and cryotherapy both cause focal temperature changes that cause cell death. RFA requires temperatures in the range of 50 to 100°C that are maintained for 5 to 8 minutes to ensure cell death. Conversely, cryotherapy requires temperatures of less than −40°C.[3] There are biologic differences in how tumors respond to the insult, with RFA causing immediate vascular coagulation and thrombosis, whereas cryoablation is characterized by sequential periods of vascular flow, vascular congestion, and thrombosis.[3] One postulated advantage of cryotherapy is the ability to monitor the developing ice ball in real time with ultrasonography.[13] However, practitioners of RFA argue that targeting accuracy is similarly achieved through three-dimensional imaging that confirms accurate deployment of the RFA probe(s) and real-time temperature monitoring. One potential advantage of percutaneous RFA is the ability to perform

Table 1
RFA series reporting intermediate-term and long-term outcomes

Author, Year	No. of Patients (No. of Tumors)	Follow-Up (mo)	Tumor Size (cm)	Biopsy-Proven RCC (%)	Approach	Incomplete Ablation (%)	Local Recurrence-Free Survival (%)	Metastasis-Free Survival (%)	Disease-Free Status (%)	Death From RCC (%)	Overall Survival (%)
Levinson et al,[27] 2008	18 (18)	Mean 57.4 (range 41–80)	Mean 2.1 (range 1–4)	51.6	Perc	3	79.9	100	100	CSS: 100	58.3
McDougal et al,[28] 2005	16 (20)	Mean 55	Mean 3.2	100	Perc	—	91 (4 y actual)	100	—	CSS: 100	68.7
Ferakis et al,[30] 2010	31 (39)	Mean 61 (range 36–84)	Mean 3.1 (range 1.3–7.5)	None biopsied	Perc	10	89 (5 y actuarial)	100	—	CSS: 100	5/31 deaths
Zagoria et al,[20] 2007	41 (48)	Median 56	Median 2.6 (range 0.7–8.2)	100	Perc	12	88 (5 y actuarial)	3/41 cases of metastasis	88 (5 y actuarial)	1/41 death from RCC	66 (5 y actuarial)
Tracy et al,[29] 2010 (Subgroup Analysis)	160 (179)	Mean 27 (range 1.5–90)	Mean 2.4	100	Perc and Lap	3	90 (5 y actuarial)	95 (5 y actuarial)	90 (5 y actuarial)	CSS: 99 (5 y actuarial)	85 (5 y actuarial)

Abbreviations: CSS, cancer-specific survival; Lap, laparoscopic; Perc, percutaneous.

Table 2
Cryotherapy series reporting intermediate and long-term outcomes

Author, Year	No. of Patients (No. of Tumors)	Follow-Up (mo)	Tumor Size (cm)	% Biopsy-Proven RCC	Approach	Incomplete Ablation	Local Recurrence	Metastasis-Free Survival	Disease-Free Status (%)	Death From RCC (%)	Overall Survival (%)
Weld et al,[31] 2007	31 (36)	Mean 45.7	Median 2.1 (range 0.5–4)	22/36	Lap	0	1/31	100% (3 y actual)	—	CSS: 100 3 y	—
Aron et al,[11] 2010	80 (88)	Median 93 (range 60–132)	Median 2.3 (range 0.9–5)	69%	Lap	—	5/80	6/80	81 5 y	CSS: 92 (5 y actual)	84 (5 y actual)
Guazzoni et al,[12] 2010 (subgroup analysis)	44	Mean 61.3	Median 2.14 (range 0.5–4)	100%	Lap	0	1/44	—	—	CSS: 100	93.2
Atwell et al,[35] 2010	91 (93)	Mean 26 (range 5–61)	Mean 3.4	44/93 (47%)	Lap	4%	1/93 (1%)	—	—	—	—
Tsivian et al,[21] 2010	163	Median 20 (range 6–79)	Mean 2.4	118 (72.4%)	Lap	—	7/163 (4.3%)	100%	—	—	—
Vricellas et al,[5] 2011	52 (54)	Mean 21	Mean 2.5	28/54 (52%)	Perc or Lap	2 patients (3.8%)	—	—	96.2	CSS: 100	98/1

Abbreviations: CSS, cancer-specific survival; Lap, laparoscopic; OS, overall survival; Perc, percutaneous.

salvage treatment with relative ease compared with laparoscopic-assisted approaches.[3]

There are no randomized trials comparing cryoablation and RFA, even though there are centers that perform both techniques.[16,25] One cohort study comparing percutaneous RFA and percutaneous cryoablation showed local recurrence rates of 11% (4/41) in the RFA group and 7% (4/70) in the cryoablation group, with the difference being not statistically significant. Although both techniques were used by all 5 interventional radiologists involved, the investigators offered no description of how a particular technique was selected. The possibility of significant selection bias limits the value of these results.[25]

A meta-analysis by Kunkle and colleagues[23] examined 47 studies with 1375 renal lesions treated by primarily laparoscopic cryoablation or percutaneous RFA. There were no differences in patient age, tumor size, or follow-up interval between groups. Local recurrence, defined as any radiologic enhancement after initial ablation, was higher for RFA than cryoablation (12.9% vs 5.2%, $P<.0001$). However, they also report repeat ablation rates of 8.5% versus 1.3% for RFA and cryoablation respectively. If the rate of repeat ablation is assumed to estimate the rate of primary treatment failure (radiographic enhancement immediately after ablation), it can be surmised that the local recurrence rates after satisfactory ablation are similar (RFA, 12.9–8.5 = 4.4%; cryoablation, 5.2–1.3 = 3.9%). Thus, RFA usually performed percutaneously required more secondary treatments but, when reablation was permitted, local recurrence rates were similar to LCA. Although metastasis was reported less frequently for cryoablation (1.0%) versus RFA (2.5%), this was not statistically significant ($P = .06$).

COMPARISON WITH THE GOLD STANDARD: ABLATION VERSUS SURGERY

The oncologic adequacy of RA can only be determined through comparison with PN, the gold standard for SRMs. However, direct comparison of disease-free survival rates between RA and PN series is inappropriate and likely to overestimate the efficacy of RA because PN series generally contain patients with greater mean tumor size and longer follow-up.[16,23] In contrast, overall survival is likely to favor partial nephrectomy series because they generally contain younger patients with fewer comorbidities. PN series report 5-year to 10-year oncologic efficacy of greater than 90%, and generally more than 95%. Several RFA series report similar success rates, albeit with shorter follow-up.[9,17] **Table 3** summarizes studies

that have compared outcomes of ablation and surgery.

The only RFA cohort comparison matched for tumor size included 40 patients treated by RFA and 37 by PN.[9] Local recurrence was defined as radiologic enhancement after successful ablation. There were 2 recurrences in each group. Of the patients with pathologically proven RCC, the 3-year disease-free survival rates for RFA and PN were not statistically different (91.4% vs 95.2% respectively, $P = .58$) and there were no cancer-specific deaths.

Takaki and colleagues[17] recently reported a cohort study comparing 54 patients undergoing radical nephrectomy and 51 patients undergoing RFA for T1a renal cell tumors. Cancer-specific survival was 100% in both groups at 5 years. Five-year disease-free survival was also equivalent: 98% for RFA and 95% for radical nephrectomy. These results overestimate the efficacy of RFA because only 23.5% of lesions were biopsied, whereas all surgically treated patients had pathologic confirmation of RCC.

Another 3-arm retrospective cohort study showed inferiority of RA compared with PN.[16] There were 36, 36, and 29 patients treated with laparoscopic PN, cryoablation, and RFA with differing cancer-specific survival at just 2 years of 100%, 88.5%, and 83.9% respectively. There were no metastases following PN, but 3 cases of metastasis in each of the cryoablation and RFA cohorts. Oncologic results were superior for PN despite a longer median follow-up time and mean tumor size that was 1 cm larger than the ablation cohorts (3.7 cm PN vs 2.6 cm RFA, 2.5 cm cryoablation).

Although some cohort studies suggest equivalency between RFA and surgery, there are several meta-analyses that suggest that RA has higher rates of local recurrence than surgery, which may be a reflection of the wide variability in RA success between series. Although these meta-analyses are helpful, they nevertheless deserve as much scrutiny as the individual series from which they are composed.

A meta-analysis by Kunkle and colleagues[33] included 99 studies and 6471 renal masses, of which 5037 were treated by PN, 496 by cryoablation, 607 by RFA, and 331 by active surveillance. Local recurrence was defined as any radiologic enhancement after initial therapy. PN had the lowest rate of local recurrence (2.6%) compared with cryoablation (4.6%) and RFA (11.7%), despite tumors in the PN group being larger (3.26 vs 2.69 vs 2.56 cm) with longer follow-up (54 vs 16.4 vs 18.3 months) than RFA and cryoablation respectively. Compared with PN, multivariable analysis

Table 3
RA versus surgery

Author, Year	Comparison	Study Design	No. of Patients	No. of Tumors	Follow-Up (mo)	Tumor Size (cm)	Biopsy-Proven RCC (%)	Local Recurrence (%)	Survival (%)
Turna et al,[16] 2009	LPN vs Cryo vs RFA	Cohort	101	LPN, 36 Cryo, 36 RFA, 29	Median LPN: 42.5 Cryo: 24 RFA: 14	Mean LPN 3.7 Cryo 2.5 RFA 2.6	LPN, 63.8 Cryo, 73.3 RFA, 82.8	DFS: LPN, 100 Cryo, 69.6 RFA, 33.2 ($P<.0001$) No. of patients with mets: LPN, 0 Cryo, 3 RFA, 3	2-y CSS: LPN, 100 Cryo, 88.5 RFA, 83.9 2-y OS: LPN, 91.2 Cryo, 88.5 RFA, 83.9
Stern et al,[9] 2007	PN vs RFA	Cohort study, matched for tumor size	77	PN, 37 RFA, 40	Mean (range) PN, 47 (24–93) RFA, 30 (18–42)	Mean PN, 2.43 RFA, 2.41	PN, 89 RFA, 81	3-y LRFS: PN, 95.2 RFA, 91.4 3 y DFS, PN, 95.8 RFA, 93.4	3y CSS: PN, 100 RFA, 100
Takaki et al,[17] 2010	RN vs PN vs RFA	Cohort	115	RN, 54 PN, 10 RFA, 51	Mean RN, 40.9 PN, 26 RFA, 34	Mean RN, 2.8 PN, 1.9 RFA, 2.4	RN, 100 PN, 100 RFA, only 23.5 had biopsy	DFS: RN 95 (5 y) PN, 75 (3 y) RFA, 98 (5 y)	CSS: 100 all groups OS: RN, 100 (5 y) PN, 100 (5 y) RFA, 75 (5 y)
Klatte et al,[34] 2011	PN vs LCA	Meta-analysis 55 studies	6642	PN, 5379 LCA, 1406	Mean PN, 57.3 LCA, 29.3	Mean PN, 3.0 LCA, 2.4	PN, 87.6 LCA, 59.5	Local recurrence (%): PN, 1.9 LCA, 8.5 ($P<.001$) Distant metastasis: PN, 1.9 LCA, 1.1 ($P = .126$)	—
Kunkle et al,[33] 2008	PN vs Cryo vs RFA vs AS	Meta-analysis 99 studies	6471	PN, 5037 Cryo, 496 RFA, 607 AS, 331	Mean LPN, 54 Cryo, 18.3 RFA, 16.4 AS, 33.3	Mean LPN, 3.4 Cryo, 2.56 RFA, 2.69 AS, 3.04	LPN, 87.6 Cryo, 75.8 RFA, 88.3 AS, 91 (of cases with available pathology)	Local recurrence (%): PN, 2.6 Cryo, 4.6 RFA, 11.7 AS, rate of metastasis not statistically different	CSS not statistically different

Abbreviations: AS, active surveillance; Cryo, cryoablation; CSS, cancer specific survival; DFS, disease free survival; LCA, laparoscopic cryoablation; LPN, laparoscopic partial nephrectomy; LRFS, local recurrence free survival; Mets, metastases; PN, partial nephrectomy; RN, radical nephrectomy; RFA, radiofrequency ablation.

revealed statistically significant relative risks of local recurrence of 7.45 for cryoablation and 18.23 for RFA. Cancer-specific survival rates were high and similar across all modalities, which may, in part, result from the lack of long-term follow-up at the time of the analysis.

Another recent meta-analysis comparing laparoscopic cryoablation (LCA) with PN also showed the ablation cohort to be inferior.[34] Fifty-five series with 6785 SRMs were included. The LCA cohort had a lower mean tumor size (2.4 vs 3.0 cm; $P<.001$) and shorter mean follow-up duration (29.3 vs 57.3 months; $P<.001$). Local tumor progression rates were 8.5% versus 1.9% ($P<.001$), corresponding with a nearly 5-fold increased risk of recurrence in the LCA group. No difference in rate of metastasis was detected between LCA and PN (1.1% vs 1.9% respectively, $P = .126$).

FUTURE STUDIES

Local recurrence rates seem to be higher in patients treated with RA compared with surgery. However, local recurrences might be adequately salvaged when identified early by follow-up imaging, causing no effect on cancer-specific survival, which is arguably the most important patient outcome. The current evidence, although subject to bias and limited follow-up, suggests similarity in rates of metastasis-free and cancer-specific survival across all treatment modalities. The AUA "Guideline for Management of Clinical Stage 1 Renal Mass," for example, performed a meta-analysis in 2009 that calculated both metastatic recurrence-free survival and cancer-specific survival to be greater than 95% for each of active surveillance, cryoablation, RFA, and PN.[10] Longer follow-up with larger series is required to attain more events and allow a more accurate comparison of cancer-specific survival. If local recurrences after ablation can be salvaged and long-term survival is equivalent, ablation may become more acceptable to young healthy patients as a first-line therapy. For the moment, the largest RA series contain fewer than 200 patients, with few studies reaching a minimum follow-up of 5 years.

There are no randomized controlled studies that can help to eliminate the confounding variables already discussed. A preliminary small randomized trial comparing cryoablation with RFA has been registered. Such a comparison would ideally use the same approach (laparoscopic or percutaneous) and is warranted because superiority has not yet been established between RFA and cryoablation. Although randomized trials comparing ablation

with surgery would be informative, differing local recurrence rates and the vast differences in treatment approach would make ethics approval and patient enrollment challenging. Nevertheless, the onus is on proponents of RA to establish its role in comparison with surgery. Evidence for this is likely best obtained through larger cohort studies matched for tumor size and location. In these comparative studies, lack of a statistically significant difference is only meaningful when the study has been powered sufficiently to detect a small difference (ie, 5% or less).

SUMMARY

Long-term oncologic efficacy of RFA and cryoablation are likely equivalent. RA seems to be inferior to PN because of higher local recurrence rates. Cancer-specific survival seems to be similar across treatment modalities, although this may simply reflect an indolent natural history of the targeted SRMs. Known predictors of long-term oncologic success following RA include tumor size and location. Other factors that likely contribute to success include differences in technique and experience between centers. Outcomes of RA are more prone to technical quality than surgery because surgical specimens provide histologic confirmation of margin status, whereas ablative techniques rely on cross-sectional imaging. Several individual series report RA success rates that approach the success seen in PN series. With improving techniques and longer follow-up, RA may prove to be a reasonable treatment alternative for SRMs in a select group of healthy patients wishing to avoid surgical therapy.

REFERENCES

1. Gill IS, Novick AC, Soble JJ, et al. Laparoscopic renal cryoablation: initial clinical series. Urology 1998;52:543–51.
2. Zlotta AR, Wildschutz T, Raviv G, et al. Radiofrequency interstitial tumor ablation (RITA) is a possible new modality for treatment of renal cancer: ex vivo and in vivo experience. J Endourol 1997;11:251–8.
3. Karam JA, Ahrar K, Matin SF. Ablation of kidney tumors. Surg Oncol Clin North Am 2011;20:341–53, viii.
4. Cutress ML, Ratan HL, Williams ST, et al. Update on the management of T1 renal cortical tumours. BJU Int 2010;106:1130–6.
5. Vricella GJ, Haaga JR, Adler BL, et al. Percutaneous cryoablation of renal masses: impact of patient selection and treatment parameters on outcomes. Urology 2011;77:649–54.

6. Desai MM, Aron M, Gill IS. Laparoscopic partial nephrectomy versus laparoscopic cryoablation for the small renal tumor. Urology 2005;66:23–8.

7. Raman JD, Raj GV, Lucas SM, et al. Renal functional outcomes for tumours in a solitary kidney managed by ablative or extirpative techniques. BJU Int 2010; 105:496–500.

8. Graversen JA, Mues AC, Landman J. Laparoscopic ablation of renal neoplasms. J Endourol 2011;25: 187–94.

9. Stern JM, Svatek R, Park S, et al. Intermediate comparison of partial nephrectomy and radiofrequency ablation for clinical T1a renal tumours. BJU Int 2007;100:287–90.

10. Campbell SC, Novick AC, Belldegrun A, et al. Guideline for management of the clinical T1 renal mass. J Urol 2009;182:1271–9.

11. Aron M, Kamoi K, Remer E, et al. Laparoscopic renal cryoablation: 8-year, single surgeon outcomes. J Urol 2010;183:889–95.

12. Guazzoni G, Cestari A, Buffi N, et al. Oncologic results of laparoscopic renal cryoablation for clinical T1a tumors: 8 years of experience in a single institution. Urology 2010;76:624–9.

13. Raman JD, Hall DW, Cadeddu JA. Renal ablative therapy: radiofrequency ablation and cryoablation. J Surg Oncol 2009;100:639–44.

14. Davenport MS, Caoili EM, Cohan RH, et al. MRI and CT characteristics of successfully ablated renal masses: imaging surveillance after radiofrequency ablation. AJR Am J Roentgenol 2009;192:1571–8.

15. Raman JD, Stern JM, Zeltser I, et al. Absence of viable renal carcinoma in biopsies performed more than 1 year following radio frequency ablation confirms reliability of axial imaging. J Urol 2008;179:2142–5.

16. Turna B, Kaouk JH, Frota R, et al. Minimally invasive nephron sparing management for renal tumors in solitary kidneys. J Urol 2009;182:2150–7.

17. Takaki H, Yamakado K, Soga N, et al. Midterm results of radiofrequency ablation versus nephrectomy for T1a renal cell carcinoma. Jpn J Radiol 2010;28:460–8.

18. Breen DJ, Rutherford EE, Stedman B, et al. Management of renal tumors by image-guided radiofrequency ablation: experience in 105 tumors. Cardiovasc Intervent Radiol 2007;30:936–42.

19. Gervais DA, Arellano RS, McGovern FJ, et al. Radiofrequency ablation of renal cell carcinoma: part 2, lessons learned with ablation of 100 tumors. AJR Am J Roentgenol 2005;185:72–80.

20. Zagoria RJ, Traver MA, Werle DM, et al. Oncologic efficacy of CT-guided percutaneous radiofrequency ablation of renal cell carcinomas. AJR Am J Roentgenol 2007;189:429–36.

21. Tsivian M, Lyne JC, Mayes JM, et al. Tumor size and endophytic growth pattern affect recurrence rates after laparoscopic renal cryoablation. Urology 2010; 75:307–10.

22. Hegarty NJ, Gill IS, Desai MM, et al. Probe-ablative nephron-sparing surgery: cryoablation versus radiofrequency ablation. Urology 2006;68:7–13.

23. Kunkle DA, Uzzo RG. Cryoablation or radiofrequency ablation of the small renal mass: a meta-analysis. Cancer 2008;113:2671–80.

24. Gupta A, Raman JD, Leveillee RJ, et al. General anesthesia and contrast-enhanced computed tomography to optimize renal percutaneous radiofrequency ablation: multi-institutional intermediate-term results. J Endourol 2009;23:1099–105.

25. Pirasteh A, Snyder L, Boncher N, et al. Cryoablation vs. radiofrequency ablation for small renal masses. Acad Radiol 2011;18:97–100.

26. Castle SM, Gorbatiy V, Ekwenna O, et al. Laparoscopic and image-guided radiofrequency ablation of renal tumors: patient selection and outcomes. Curr Urol Rep 2011;12:100–6.

27. Levinson AW, Su LM, Agarwal D, et al. Long-term oncological and overall outcomes of percutaneous radio frequency ablation in high risk surgical patients with a solitary small renal mass. J Urol 2008;180:499–504 [discussion: 504].

28. McDougal WS, Gervais DA, McGovern FJ, et al. Long-term followup of patients with renal cell carcinoma treated with radio frequency ablation with curative intent. J Urol 2005;174:61–3.

29. Tracy CR, Raman JD, Donnally C, et al. Durable oncologic outcomes after radiofrequency ablation: experience from treating 243 small renal masses over 7.5 years. Cancer 2010;116:3135–42.

30. Ferakis N, Bouropoulos C, Granitsas T, et al. Long-term results after computed-tomography-guided percutaneous radiofrequency ablation for small renal tumors. J Endourol 2010;24:1909–13.

31. Weld KJ, Figenshau RS, Venkatesh R, et al. Laparoscopic cryoablation for small renal masses: three-year follow-up. Urology 2007;69:448–51.

32. Davol PE, Fulmer BR, Rukstalis DB. Long-term results of cryoablation for renal cancer and complex renal masses. Urology 2006;68:2–6.

33. Kunkle DA, Egleston BL, Uzzo RG. Excise, ablate or observe: the small renal mass dilemma–a meta-analysis and review. J Urol 2008;179:1227–33 [discussion: 1233–4].

34. Klatte T, Grubmuller B, Waldert M, et al. Laparoscopic cryoablation versus partial nephrectomy for the treatment of small renal masses: systematic review and cumulative analysis of observational studies. Eur Urol 2011;60:435–43.

35. Atwell TD, Callstrom MR, Farrell MA, et al. Percutaneous renal cryoablation: local control at mean 26 months of followup. J Urol 2010;184:1291–5.

The Influence of Surgical Approach to the Renal Mass on Renal Function

Brian R. Lane, MD, PhD[a,b,c],*, Christopher M. Whelan, MD[a,b]

KEYWORDS

- Kidney neoplasms • Nephrectomy • Partial nephrectomy
- Chronic kidney disease • Renal function

The National Kidney Foundation estimates that 26 million Americans are living with chronic kidney disease (CKD).[1] The high prevalence of obesity, heart disease, hypertension, and diabetes places millions more at risk for developing CKD.[1] When counseling patients with a newly diagnosed renal mass, treatment effect on renal function should always be a central part of the discussion.[2] Although long-term sufficient renal function is routine in screened kidney donors, CKD is present in more than 30% of patients with a newly diagnosed renal mass and develops in most patients who undergo radical nephrectomy (RN) and a portion of those who undergo nephron-sparing approaches.[3,4] Although radical surgery for kidney cancer can cure one disease (cancer), it can often lead to another (CKD) that may be just as concerning.

The average 60-year-old patient can expect to live another 21 years, whereas a 60-year-old person on dialysis has an average of only 4.6 years left to live.[1] However, the negative impact of decreasing renal function begins in patients long before they require renal replacement therapy. Patients with moderate to severe CKD (glomerular filtration rates [GFRs], 15–60 mL/min/1.73 m^2) have dose-related increases in cardiovascular events.[5] Routinely, the assessment of renal function has relied on whether the serum creatinine (sCr) levels fall within the normal range.[6] However, given the variability of sCr with differences in gender, muscle mass, and hydration status, this approach is frequently misleading. Small changes in sCr values can signify large changes in global renal function, and an sCr value in the normal range may fail to detect a clinically significant decline in renal function. For example, a normal sCr level of 1.2 mg/dL in a thin, inactive, elderly woman can signify stage 3, or even stage 4, CKD. Estimates of GFR that rely on sCr and other clinical factors (age, gender, race) are more accurate than sCr alone, and such estimates indicate that CKD is much more common than previously recognized.[6] Patients with a GFR less than 45 are 11 times more likely to experience a major cardiovascular event than those with normal renal function.[5] Herein, the authors review the effect of the surgical approach on renal function for patients presenting with a renal mass.

TREATMENT OPTIONS FOR PATIENTS WITH LOCALIZED KIDNEY TUMORS

RN was developed as the standard treatment of kidney tumors in the latter half of the twentieth century. In 1969, Robson reported the outcomes of 88 patients who underwent RN (described as

[a] Spectrum Health, 100 Michigan Street NE, Grand Rapids, MI 49503, USA
[b] Department of Surgery, Michigan State University College of Human Medicine, 15 Michigan Street NE, Grand Rapids, MI 49503, USA
[c] Labaratories of Computational Biology and Genetic Epidemiology, Van Andel Research Institute, 333 Bostwick Avenue NE, Grand Rapids, MI 49503, USA
* Corresponding author. Urology Division, Spectrum Health Medical Group, 4069 Lake Drive, Suite 313, Grand Rapids, MI 49546.
E-mail address: brian.lane@spectrumhealth.org

Urol Clin N Am 39 (2012) 191–198
doi:10.1016/j.ucl.2012.01.007
0094-0143/12/$ – see front matter © 2012 Elsevier Inc. All rights reserved.

the perifascial resection of the kidney along with the perirenal fat, ipsilateral adrenal gland, and regional lymph nodes). He found a survival rate of 65% for patients with tumors confined within the Gerota fascia. This technique represented a significant survival benefit over other treatments and became the standard approach to renal tumors for the next 20 years. Laparoscopic RN (LRN) was introduced in 1991 and has since been readily adopted as a less invasive approach. Transperitoneal, retroperitoneal, robot-assisted, and hand-assisted LRN techniques are all proven techniques that are selected primarily based on surgeon experience and preference. In appropriately selected patients, LRN has comparable oncologic efficacy and improved morbidity and recovery compared with open RN (ORN). In the 1980s and 1990s, open partial nephrectomy (OPN) began emerging in academic centers as an option for patients with an absolute need to preserve renal parenchyma. Patients with bilateral renal tumors, tumors in a solitary functioning kidney, and/or chronic renal failure were considered candidates. The goal for such patients was avoidance of dialysis, even if oncologic efficacy was somewhat compromised. The concept of elective partial nephrectomy (PN) met resistance in the surgical community based on an increased potential for local recurrence. In addition, the deleterious cardiovascular effects of CKD in patients not yet requiring dialysis were still unknown at this time. As the concept of the risks associated with CKD expanded throughout the surgical community and the oncologic efficacy of PN became established, the role of elective PN for small renal masses (SRMs) of sizes less than 4 cm began to expand. Building off of techniques used for LRN and OPN, Gill and others[7] pioneered the development of laparoscopic PN (LPN) as a minimally invasive, nephron-sparing approach for the management of SRMs. The addition of robotics as a tool for LPN is expanding the application of this surgery in appropriately selected patients.[8] Thermal ablation (TA) technologies, such as cryoablation (CA) and radiofrequency ablation (RFA), are alternative minimally invasive, nephron-sparing treatments of SRMs. Surveillance of renal tumors is also an option, particularly for patients with SRMs and major comorbidities in whom avoidance of the risks of intervention may be preferable to the small risk of cancer progression. With so many options for kidney tumors, particularly for SRMs, patients and clinicians must be well informed to make decisions that are associated with the most favorable outcomes. The importance of avoiding CKD through the appropriate use of nephron-sparing approaches

is gaining ground in the urologic surgical community and is reflected in the recent release of clinical guidelines for the management of SRMs by the American Urologic Association (AUA) and European Association of Urology.[9,10]

AUA GUIDELINES

The natural history of renal tumors that are smaller than 7 cm is variable; only 20% to 30% demonstrate aggressive features, and up to 20% are benign.[11,12] However, the most recently published summary of current practice pattern in the United States shows that 65% of kidney cancers are treated with RN and 35% with PN.[13] These data, coupled with the growing emphasis on the importance of preserving renal function, prompted the AUA to release clinical guidelines to address the management of clinical stage 1 renal masses.[9] Recommendations for 4 index patients were discussed, including patients with tumors that are less than 4 cm or 4 to 7 cm in size and those who are healthy or with major comorbidities and increased surgical risk. RN and PN were both recommended as standard for 3 index patients. For index patient 4 (medical comorbidities, increased surgical risk, and a tumor of 4–7 cm), RN was thought to be "standard" with "complete surgical excision by PN… a recommended modality when there is a need to preserve renal function, although it can be associated with increased urologic morbidity."[9] TA and active surveillance (AS) were discussed as options for healthy patients and were recommended particularly in patients with increased surgical risk. Throughout these guidelines, a discussion of the risks and benefits of each approach was emphasized, given the complexity of the landscape for treatment of SRMs and the significant impact of treatment approach on various outcomes.

THE APPLICABILITY OF OUTCOMES OF DONOR NEPHRECTOMY

Until recently, urologists used the satisfactory renal functional outcomes in kidney donors to counsel patients that removal of one kidney would not lead to long-term problems. Ibrahim and colleagues[14] published the long-term consequences of kidney donation in a cohort of 3698 healthy donors, finding no significant differences in the development of end-stage renal disease or overall survival compared with matched controls. Although these data might encourage patients and clinicians to suspect that RN for cancer may not carry significant risks attributable to the loss of renal function, caution should be exercised because patients with renal cancer are different from healthy screened donors. The mean age of the donor population is 41 years, whereas the mean age is greater than 60 years for patients who present with a renal mass. Smoking, obesity, and hypertension are established risk factors for the development of renal cell carcinoma and are more prevalent in patients with a renal mass. Bijol and colleagues[15] reviewed a series of nephrectomy specimens for patients undergoing RN. Apart from the tumor within the normal part of the kidney, 62% of the specimens showed microscopic signs of renal disease. Huang and associates[3] reported on 662 patients with SRM, a normal contralateral kidney, and normal sCr levels. Even in these patients, 26% had preexisting CKD, as evidenced by a GFR less than 60 using the MDRD (modification of diet in renal disease) formula.[3] Although long-term sufficient renal function is routine in screened kidney donors, CKD develops in between 50% and 65% of patients after RN.[3,4] Indeed, radical surgery can often substitute one disease for another.

RADICAL NEPHRECTOMY

RN remains the treatment of choice for large (>7 cm) and locally advanced renal tumors, which are the most lethal of genitourinary malignancies.[16] TA and surveillance are inadequate for prevention of cancer progression in these situations. For such tumors, preservation of sufficient functioning renal parenchyma can often not be possible with PN. The problem with RN is that it is often overused and invariably increases the risk for the development of CKD when compared with these other approaches.[3,13] LRN can be swiftly performed and can provide the patient with minimal morbidity and a fast recovery, but the long-term effects of this approach can be significant. For clinical stage T1 tumors, PN is associated with a higher rate of urologic complications in the short term but improved early and late renal functional outcomes when compared with RN.[9] Huang and colleagues[3] found that 65% of patients undergoing RN developed stage 3 or higher CKD (estimated GFR <60 mL/min/1.73 m^2) within 3 years of RN. In addition, patients undergoing RN were 3.8 times more likely to develop stage 3 CKD than those undergoing PN. Although most of these patients will never require dialysis, CKD has a dose-related relationship with cardiovascular events and is a powerful contributor to patient mortality.[5] The negative impact of RN-induced CKD has been confirmed in several subsequent studies.[17,18]

Although these data should push surgeons to consider PN for SRMs, RN remains the gold standard approach for larger renal masses. The benefits of renal preservation must be weighed against sound oncologic principles. Indeed, the oncologic importance of a complete wide excision for larger tumors is highlighted by the fact that up to 25% have involvement of the perinephric fat.[16] Before performing RN, the surgeon should evaluate each patient's risk for developing CKD after surgery. A GFR estimation equation, such as the MDRD study equation or the newer CKD-EPI (Chronic Kidney Disease Epidemiology Collaboration) study equations, should be used before surgery.[6] Assuming 2 radiographically and functionally similar kidneys, an approximately 35% decline in GFR can be expected with unilateral RN (**Table 1**).[4] More accurate prediction tools, or nomograms, have also been developed and can be useful for patient counseling.[19] Patients should be counseled regarding the risks of CKD, along with its associated cardiovascular and other complications. Patients found to be at significant risk of becoming dialysis dependent should see a nephrologist for preoperative counseling.[20] In select cases, a dialysis catheter can be placed at the time of surgery or in the immediate postoperative period.

Whether completed in an open or a laparoscopic manner, basic surgical principles should be followed to maintain and protect the unaffected kidney during RN. Patients at risk for cardiopulmonary complications should be screened by a cardiologist before surgery. To reduce the risk of infection and sepsis, preoperative urinalysis and culture results should be obtained and appropriate prophylactic (or therapeutic) antibiotic used. Appropriate patient positioning and the avoidance of prolonged surgery can minimize the risks of rhabdomyolysis and its deleterious effect on kidney function. Adequate exposure and an understanding of the patient's renal vascular anatomy are paramount to minimize blood loss and risk of intraoperative hypotension. Some investigators have used preoperative embolization to try to minimize intraoperative hemorrhage, but Subramanian and colleagues[21] have recently shown that this maneuver may have the opposite effect. Laparoscopic techniques themselves, by establishment of pneumoperitoneum and reduction of venous bleeding, may lessen the impact of surgery on early renal function as well.[16] Therefore, when a nephron-sparing approach is not feasible, RN is the treatment of choice. The decreased renal function attributable to nephron loss is generally offset by the significant oncologic benefit of the surgery.

Table 1
Summary of renal functional changes according to type of management for renal mass (numerical values in percentages)

Surgery	Ipsilateral Parenchyma Removed (%)	Total Parenchyma Preserved (%)	Median Loss of Renal Function (%)	% Developing New-onset CKD (GFR <45)
RN	100	Approximately 50	35[3,4]	35–43[3,4]
PN with extended ischemia (>30 min)	25 (15–60)[2]	Approximately 70–90	19[4]	19[4]
PN with regional hypothermia	20 (15–40)[3]	Approximately 75–92	11[30]	10[30]
PN with limited ischemia (<30 min)	20 (10–40)[2,3]	Approximately 80–95	12[4,30]	10[4,30]
PN without ischemia	10 (0–20)[3]	Approximately 90–100	5–10[30,35]	7[30]
TA	0	Approximately 90–100	0–10[55,56,58]	NA
AS	0	100	0–5[63,64]	NA

References from main text.
Abbreviation: NA, not available.

PARTIAL NEPHRECTOMY

When compared with RN, PN always provides better renal functional outcomes in similar patients (see **Table 1**).[4] Although it would be expected that this benefit would disappear for tumors large enough and/or extending deep enough into the renal hilum, such outcomes have not yet been reported.[4,22] In fact, several series report on successful use of PN for tumors larger than 7 cm or with renal vein thrombus.[22–25] This collective experience has led some investigators to conclude that preservable parenchyma, and not tumor size, should be the main determinant of the feasibility of PN.[26]

Initial investigations into the factors predicting renal function after PN revealed that lower preoperative GFR, solitary kidney, lesser parenchymal preservation, longer warm ischemic interval, larger tumor size, and older age are independent predictors of reduced postoperative GFR.[27] Subsequent data specifically regarding patients undergoing PN in a solitary kidney suggested an increase of 5% to 6% in the risk of acute kidney injury or CKD with each additional minute of warm ischemia.[28] Several other studies also suggested a strong correlation between ischemia time and loss of renal function, leading to the concept that every minute counts. The authors' subsequent work has demonstrated that although the type and duration of renal ischemia may be the strongest modifiable risk factors for decreased renal function after PN, factors that are for the most part nonmodifiable, the preoperative GFR and the amount of spared parenchyma, that is, quality and quantity of the spared parenchyma, play a predominant role.[29] Improved understanding of this complex topic has recently been provided by a 4-center study of open PN under either warm (n = 360) or cold (n = 300) ischemia in patients with solitary kidneys.[29] Despite 23 minutes longer ischemia during PN with cold ischemia (median, 45 minutes) than PN with warm ischemia (median, 22 min), similar decreases in postoperative GFR (21% vs 22%) and ultimate GFR (10% vs 9%) were observed, confirming a protective effect of hypothermia.[29] Reasons for longer ischemia with the hypothermic cases were multifactorial, including the wait for 10 to 15 minutes that had been routinely practiced, selection biases, the cumbersome nature of ice-slush usage, and/or relief of the sense of urgency because of hypothermia.[29] Importantly, factors that strongly correlated with longer ischemic time included not only hypothermia but also the amount of spared parenchyma (P<.0001). Simpler cases, in which the amount of spared parenchyma was greatest, were performed with the shortest ischemic times. Ischemia time seems to serve as a correlate of complexity in this (and other) series of patients. Final multivariate analysis of this dataset suggested that preoperative GFR and percentage of parenchyma preserved stood out as strongly predictive of early and ultimate renal function (each P<.0001). Ischemia time was not associated with renal function in this particular study

$(P = .5)$.[29] Sixty-eight percent of patients in this series underwent PN under hypothermic conditions or with 20 minutes or less of warm ischemia and only 12% of warm ischemic intervals exceeded 30 minutes, consistent with the high standards for conventional PN at these centers of excellence.[29] This study suggests that if the ischemic interval is kept short or if hypothermia is applied, ultimate loss of function due to ischemic injury pales in comparison to the quantity and quality of kidney preserved. These data are confirmed by analysis of outcomes in the 2-kidney model, in which nonischemic PN, PN under cold ischemia, and PN under warm ischemia up to 20 minutes were associated with similar renal functional outcomes.[30] A reanalysis of the populations of patients from the Cleveland Clinic and Mayo Clinic study on PN in a solitary kidney under warm ischemia (and with a wider range of intervals) indicated that warm ischemia time retained some predictive value.[28,31] Although the quantity and quality of preserved parenchyma stood out as the predominant predictors of ultimate renal function after PN, the subgroup of patients with warm ischemic interval greater than 25 minutes was at about a 2-fold increased risk for de novo severe CKD.[31]

The use of a minimally invasive approach to PN, including LPN and robot-assisted LPN, does not seem to have an impact on renal function when compared with OPN.[9,27,32] Although initial series of LPN reported longer warm ischemia times than used with OPN and infrequently used hypothermia, more recent reports indicate that LPN can be performed with short ischemic intervals, selective clamping of tertiary or quaternary renal arterial branches, or off clamp.[33–35] In addition, more recent reports now indicate that robot-assisted LPN can be performed with a lesser impact on renal function than traditional LPN, in part because of these same technical variations.[36–41]

To optimize PN, the authors believe that careful presurgical planning and precision during intrarenal dissection may maximize the amount of preserved parenchyma, while still achieving negative margins, and careful reconstruction can minimize ischemic areas adjacent to the renorrhaphy. One potential way to reduce the amount of healthy parenchyma resected or devascularized is using neoadjuvant systemic therapy to decrease tumor volume. Initial investigations have suggested that various agents, such as sunitinib, sorafenib, temsirolimus, and others, can produce partial reductions in tumor volume and that PN is feasible after these treatments.[42] However, the oncologic efficacy and overall impact of such treatments remain to be determined and should be done in the context of clinical trials. According to the authors, more precise determination of renal damage on the ipsilateral kidney enables more precise evaluation of the causes of such damage. Further advances in radiographic evaluation of renal damage using functional studies, such as technetium renal scintigraphy[43] and functional magnetic resonance imaging[44] or molecular markers, such as KIM-1 and N-GAL,[45] may allow for investigations into early interventions to improve long-term renal functional outcomes. Clearly, this is a fruitful field for subsequent clinical and translational research.

THERMAL ABLATION

TA techniques, such as CA and RFA, are alternative minimally invasive, nephron-sparing treatments of SRMs. These techniques can be performed in a percutaneous or laparoscopic manner and do not require dissection and clamping of the renal hilum, avoiding ischemic insult to the ipsilateral renal unit.[46,47] Several clinical series indicate that TA may offer the potential for reduced morbidity and recovery compared with ORN, OPN, LRN, and LPN.[9,48–53] However, the data supporting the oncologic efficacy of TA are not as robust as OPN or LRN, and meta-analyses suggest decreased efficacy compared with extirpative approaches.[52,54] Kunkle and Uzzo[52] performed a comparative meta-analysis to evaluate CA and RFA as primary treatments of SRMs. Here, the data favored CA for local tumor control and for potential lower risk of metastatic progression compared with RFA.

Comparisons of renal functional outcomes in patients undergoing TA or PN for tumor in a solitary kidney reveal essentially no difference between the techniques, despite the use of ischemia with some PNs.[55–59] A group at the Mayo clinic recently compared the renal function outcomes in patients with solitary kidneys undergoing percutaneous TA with that in those who underwent PN.[57] At the 3-month follow-up, the investigators noted no significant difference in renal function between both the groups.[57] Despite perceived differences in oncologic efficacy, there seems to be no difference in the preservation of renal function, using any ablative or extirpative nephron-sparing technique to date. These findings again highlight the importance of the quantity and quality of preserved parenchyma as the key determinant of ultimate renal function.

ACTIVE SURVEILLANCE

The relationship between CKD and mortality has prompted researchers to consider the role of AS in patients with SRMs. Reviews from multiple institutions show that the growth rate of SRMs is slow, approximately 2.8 mm per year, with a metastasis rate of 1.2%.[54,60–63] Although promising, the data on AS remain in its early stages because most series report surveillance of no more than 2 to 3 years with growth rates that are calculated retrospectively. Nonetheless, in patients who are at high surgical risk, AS is a viable option with serial renal imaging performed at 6- to 12-month intervals. Lane and colleagues[64] recently reported on a series of 537 patients who were 75 years or older, of whom 432 underwent active surgical management, including RN and nephron-sparing approaches. With a mean follow-up of 4 years, the investigators found that active treatment did not confer a statistically significant survival benefit compared with AS (hazard ratio [nephron-sparing interventions vs AS], 0.67; 95% confidence interval, 0.42–1.05; $P = .22$).[64] The oncologic benefits of active treatment may have been offset by the lost renal function with these approaches. As might be expected, renal function remained reasonably stable during the period of surveillance in this and more recent studies.[64,65] In appropriately selected patients, AS is the most minimally invasive, nephron-sparing, and function-preserving option in the management of SRMs.

SUMMARY

The surgical approach to the renal mass continues to evolve as a more nuanced appreciation of the biology of renal masses, a more precise approach to individual patients and their tumors, and a deeper understanding of the factors influencing baseline and postoperative renal function have been developed. Tumor size and location provide the key information for the selection of surgical approach to the renal mass, particularly for SRMs. The potential morbidity of each approach, particularly the anticipated effect on renal function, should also play a central role in deciding the course of treatment (see **Table 1**). RN is appropriate when the quantity and quality of the renal remnant would be severely reduced after a kidney-sparing technique such as PN. TA and AS are also options for SRMs, particularly in individuals at increased perioperative risk. Increased use of kidney-sparing approaches in recent years is encouraging, but more work needs to be done to educate surgeons and patients on the long-term benefits of preserving renal function, particularly for patients with low-risk tumors.

REFERENCES

1. National Kidney Foundation. The facts about chronic kidney disease (CKD). Available at: http://www.kidney.org/kidneydisease/ckd/index.cfm. Accessed November 1, 2011.
2. Lane BR, Campbell SC. Management of small renal masses. AUA Update 2009;28(34):314–23.
3. Huang WC, Levey AS, Serio AM, et al. Chronic kidney disease after nephrectomy in patients with renal cortical tumours: a retrospective cohort study. Lancet Oncol 2006;7(9):735–40.
4. Lane BR, Fergany AF, Weight CJ, et al. Renal functional outcomes after partial nephrectomy with extended ischemic intervals are better than after radical nephrectomy. J Urol 2010;184(4):1286–90.
5. Go AS, Chertow GM, Fan D, et al. Chronic kidney disease and the risks of death, cardiovascular events, and hospitalization. N Engl J Med 2004;351(13):1296–305.
6. Lane BR, Poggio ED, Herts BR, et al. Renal function assessment in the era of chronic kidney disease: renewed emphasis on renal function centered patient care. J Urol 2009;182(2):435–43 [discussion: 443–4].
7. Gill IS, Desai MM, Kaouk JH, et al. Laparoscopic partial nephrectomy for renal tumor: duplicating open surgical techniques. J Urol 2002;167(2 Pt 1). 469–75 [discussion: 475–6].
8. Rogers C, Sukumar S, Gill IS. Robotic partial nephrectomy: the real benefit. Curr Opin Urol 2011;21(1):60–4.
9. Campbell SC, Novick AC, Belldegrun A, et al. Guideline for management of the clinical T1 renal mass. J Urol 2009;182(4):1271–9.
10. Ljungberg B, Cowan NC, Hanbury DC, et al. EAU guidelines on renal cell carcinoma: the 2010 update. Eur Urol 2010;58(3):398–406.
11. Frank I, Blute ML, Cheville JC, et al. Solid renal tumors: an analysis of pathological features related to tumor size. J Urol 2003;170(6 Pt 1):2217–20.
12. Lane BR, Babineau D, Kattan MW, et al. A preoperative prognostic nomogram for solid enhancing renal tumors 7 cm or less amenable to partial nephrectomy. J Urol 2007;178(2):429–34.
13. Dulabon LM, Lowrance WT, Russo P, et al. Trends in renal tumor surgery delivery within the United States. Cancer 2010;116(10):2316–21.
14. Ibrahim HN, Foley R, Tan L, et al. Long-term consequences of kidney donation. N Engl J Med 2009;360(5):459–69.
15. Bijol V, Mendez GP, Hurwitz S, et al. Evaluation of the nonneoplastic pathology in tumor nephrectomy specimens: predicting the risk of progressive renal failure. Am J Surg Pathol 2006;30(5):575–84.
16. Campbell SC, Lane BR. Malignant renal tumors. In: Wein AJ, Kavoussi LR, Novick AC, et al, editors. Cambell-Walsh urology. 10th edition. Philadelphia (PA): Saunders; 2011. p. 1413–74. Chapter 49.
17. Thompson RH, Boorjian SA, Lohse CM, et al. Radical nephrectomy for pT1a renal masses may be associated with decreased overall survival

compared with partial nephrectomy. J Urol 2008; 179(2):468–71 [discussion: 472–3].

18. Weight CJ, Larson BT, Fergany AF, et al. Nephrectomy induced chronic renal insufficiency is associated with increased risk of cardiovascular death and death from any cause in patients with localized cT1b renal masses. J Urol 2010;183(4):1317–23.

19. Sorbellini M, Kattan MW, Snyder ME, et al. Prognostic nomogram for renal insufficiency after radical or partial nephrectomy. J Urol 2006;176(2):472–6 [discussion: 476].

20. Smart NA, Titus TT. Outcomes of early versus late nephrology referral in chronic kidney disease: a systematic review. Am J Med 2011;124(11): 1073–80 e2.

21. Subramanian VS, Stephenson AJ, Goldfarb DA, et al. Utility of preoperative renal artery embolization for management of renal tumors with inferior vena caval thrombi. Urology 2009;74(1):154–9.

22. Weight CJ, Lythgoe C, Unnikrishnan R, et al. Partial nephrectomy does not compromise survival in patients with pathologic upstaging to pT2/pT3 or high-grade renal tumors compared with radical nephrectomy. Urology 2011;77(5):1142–6.

23. Breau RH, Crispen PL, Jimenez RE, et al. Outcome of stage T2 or greater renal cell cancer treated with partial nephrectomy. J Urol 2010;183(3):903–8.

24. Woldu SL, Barlow LJ, Patel T, et al. Single institutional experience with nephron-sparing surgery for pathologic stage T3bNxM0 renal cell carcinoma confined to the renal vein. Urology 2010;76(3): 639–42.

25. Kolla SB, Ercole C, Spiess PE, et al. Nephronsparing surgery for pathological stage T3b renal cell carcinoma confined to the renal vein. BJU Int 2010;106(10):1494–8.

26. Lane BR, Fergany AF, Linehan WM, et al. Should preservable parenchyma, and not tumor size, be the main determinant of the feasibility of partial nephrectomy? Urology 2010;76(3):608–9.

27. Lane BR, Babineau DC, Poggio ED, et al. Factors predicting renal functional outcome after partial nephrectomy. J Urol 2008;180(6):2363–8 [discussion: 2368–9].

28. Thompson RH, Lane BR, Lohse CM, et al. Every minute counts when the renal hilum is clamped during partial nephrectomy. Eur Urol 2010;58(3): 340–5.

29. Lane BR, Russo P, Uzzo RG, et al. Comparison of cold and warm ischemia during partial nephrectomy in 660 solitary kidneys reveals predominant role of nonmodifiable factors in determining ultimate renal function. J Urol 2011;185(2):421–7.

30. Lane BR, Gill IS, Fergany AF, et al. Limited warm ischemia during elective partial nephrectomy has only a marginal impact on renal functional outcomes. J Urol 2011;185(5):1598–603.

31. Thompson RH, Lane BR, Lohse CM, et al. Comparison of warm ischemia versus no ischemia during partial nephrectomy on a solitary kidney. Eur Urol 2010;58(3):331–6.

32. Gill IS, Kavoussi LR, Lane BR, et al. Comparison of 1,800 laparoscopic and open partial nephrectomies for single renal tumors. J Urol 2007;178(1):41–6.

33. Ukimura O, Nakamoto M, Gill IS. Three-dimensional reconstruction of renovascular-tumor anatomy to facilitate zero-ischemia partial nephrectomy. Eur Urol 2012;61(1):211–7.

34. Ng CK, Gill IS, Patil MB, et al. Anatomic renal artery branch microdissection to facilitate zeroischemia partial nephrectomy. Eur Urol 2012; 61(1):67–74.

35. Gill IS, Eisenberg MS, Aron M, et al. "Zero ischemia" partial nephrectomy: novel laparoscopic and robotic technique. Eur Urol 2011;59(1):128–34.

36. Benway BM, Bhayani SB, Rogers CG, et al. Robot assisted partial nephrectomy versus laparoscopic partial nephrectomy for renal tumors: a multi-institutional analysis of perioperative outcomes. J Urol 2009;182(3):866–72.

37. Seo IY, Choi H, Boldbaatr Y, et al. Operative outcomes of robotic partial nephrectomy: a comparison with conventional laparoscopic partial nephrectomy. Korean J Urol 2011;52(4):279–83.

38. Reyes JM, Smaldone MC, Uzzo RG, et al. Current status of robot-assisted partial nephrectomy. Curr Urol Rep 2012;13(1):24–37.

39. Pierorazio PM, Patel HD, Feng T, et al. Robotic-assisted versus traditional laparoscopic partial nephrectomy: comparison of outcomes and evaluation of learning curve. Urology 2011;78(4):813–9.

40. Kowalczyk KJ, Alemozaffar M, Hevelone ND, et al. Partial clamping of the renal artery during roboticassisted laparoscopic partial nephrectomy: technique and initial outcomes. J Endourol 2011. [Epub ahead of print].

41. Kaouk JH, Hillyer SP, Autorino R, et al. 252 robotic partial nephrectomies: evolving renorrhaphy technique and surgical outcomes at a single institution. Urology 2011;78(6):1338–44.

42. Hellenthal NJ, Underwood W, Penetrante R, et al. Prospective clinical trial of preoperative sunitinib in patients with renal cell carcinoma. J Urol 2010; 184(3):859–64.

43. Choi JD, Park JW, Choi JY, et al. Renal damage caused by warm ischaemia during laparoscopic and robot-assisted partial nephrectomy: an assessment using Tc 99m-DTPA glomerular filtration rate. Eur Urol 2010;58(6):900–5.

44. Kang S, Bruhn A, Chandarana H, et al. Pre- and post-operative measurement of single kidney function in partial nephrectomy for renal masses using magnetic resonance renography [abstract 1080]. J Urol 2010;185(4).

45. Lane BR. Molecular markers of kidney injury. Urol Oncol 2011. [Epub ahead of print].

46. Finley DS, Beck S, Box G, et al. Percutaneous and laparoscopic cryoablation of small renal masses. J Urol 2008;180(2):492–8 [discussion: 498].

47. Long CJ, Kutikov A, Canter DJ, et al. Percutaneous vs surgical cryoablation of the small renal mass: is efficacy compromised? BJU Int 2011;107(9):1376–80.

48. Matin SF, Ahrar K. Nephron-sparing probe ablative therapy: long-term outcomes. Curr Opin Urol 2008; 18(2):150–6.

49. Haber GP, Lee MC, Crouzet S, et al. Tumour in solitary kidney: laparoscopic partial nephrectomy vs laparoscopic cryoablation. BJU Int 2012;109(1):118–24.

50. Berger A, Kamoi K, Gill IS, et al. Cryoablation for renal tumors: current status. Curr Opin Urol 2009; 19(2):138–42.

51. Carraway WA, Raman JD, Cadeddu JA. Current status of renal radiofrequency ablation. Curr Opin Urol 2009;19(2):143–7.

52. Kunkle DA, Uzzo RG. Cryoablation or radiofrequency ablation of the small renal mass: a meta-analysis. Cancer 2008;113(10):2671–80.

53. Zagoria RJ, Childs DD. Update on thermal ablation of renal cell carcinoma: oncologic control, technique comparison, renal function preservation, and new modalities. Curr Urol Rep 2012;13(1):63–9.

54. Kunkle DA, Egleston BL, Uzzo RG. Excise, ablate or observe: the small renal mass dilemma—a meta-analysis and review. J Urol 2008;179(4):1227–33 [discussion: 1233–4].

55. Turna B, Kaouk JH, Frota R, et al. Minimally invasive nephron sparing management for renal tumors in solitary kidneys. J Urol 2009;182(5):2150–7.

56. Raman JD, Raj GV, Lucas SM, et al. Renal functional outcomes for tumours in a solitary kidney managed by ablative or extirpative techniques. BJU Int 2010; 105(4):496–500.

57. Mitchell CR, Atwell TD, Weisbrod AJ, et al. Renal function outcomes in patients treated with partial nephrectomy versus percutaneous ablation for renal tumors in a solitary kidney. J Urol 2011;186(5):1786–90.

58. Mues AC, Okhunov Z, Haramis G, et al. Comparison of percutaneous and laparoscopic renal cryoablation for small (<3.0 cm) renal masses. J Endourol 2010;24(7):1097–100.

59. Pettus JA, Werle DM, Saunders W, et al. Percutaneous radiofrequency ablation does not affect glomerular filtration rate. J Endourol 2010;24(10): 1687–91.

60. Smaldone MC, Kutikov A, Egleston BL, et al. Small renal masses progressing to metastases under active surveillance: a systematic review and pooled analysis. Cancer 2011. [Epub ahead of print].

61. Crispen PL, Viterbo R, Boorjian SA, et al. Natural history, growth kinetics, and outcomes of untreated clinically localized renal tumors under active surveillance. Cancer 2009;115(13):2844–52.

62. Abouassaly R, Lane BR, Novick AC. Active surveillance of renal masses in elderly patients. J Urol 2008;180(2):505–8 [discussion: 508–9].

63. Crispen PL, Wong YN, Greenberg RE, et al. Predicting growth of solid renal masses under active surveillance. Urol Oncol 2008;26(5):555–9.

64. Lane BR, Abouassaly R, Gao T, et al. Active treatment of localized renal tumors may not impact overall survival in patients aged 75 years or older. Cancer 2010;116(13):3119–26.

65. Almatur A, Margel D, Finelli T, et al. Natural history of renal function in untreated kidney cancer [abstract 137]. Urol Onc. Presented at SUO meeting. Bethesda (MD), December 5, 2011.

Partial Nephrectomy: Contemporary Outcomes, Candidate Selection, and Surgical Approach

Emil Kheterpal, MD[a], Samir S. Taneja, MD[b],*

KEYWORDS

- Renal cell carcinoma • Partial nephrectomy • Outcomes
- Candidate selection • Renal ischemia • Technique

Partial nephrectomy (PN) has historically been used in urology for the treatment of benign processes of the kidney such as stone disease, nonfunction within a duplicated moiety, trauma, and infection. In the past 20 years, the major application of PN has been the treatment of localized renal tumors as an alternative to RN. Initially, indications were absolute, including patients with solitary kidney and bilateral tumors. With time, indications broadened based upon risk factors for kidney disease, and eventually elective PN was performed for tumors less than 4 cm in patients with normal kidney function and contralateral kidney. The safety of this approach has been proven through long-term follow-up, thereby allowing broadened indications for tumors larger than 4 cm. Today most renal cortical lesions are detected incidentally due to widespread use of medical imaging. Despite the long history and proven efficacy of radical nephrectomy (RN) in treating kidney cancer, the downward stage migration of renal cell carcinoma (RCC) and recent data demonstrating an increased risk of chronic kidney disease (CKD) with RN has called into question the use of RN as the treatment of choice in patients with newly diagnosed kidney tumors.[1]

OUTCOMES: ONCOLOGIC, COMPLICATIONS, RENAL FUNCTION

Oncologic Outcomes of PN

PN for renal tumor balances complete resection of the tumor-bearing portion of the kidney while preserving as much normal renal parenchyma as possible.[1] Advantages of PN are the preservation of renal function, a reduced risk of future CKD, and avoidance of overtreatment of benign renal masses by nephrectomy.[2] Despite studies demonstrating the importance of renal preservation in regard to renal function, local cancer control is still the primary goal of any cancer surgery, and acceptable oncologic efficacy must be demonstrated before PN can be accepted as a viable alternative to RN in an elective setting.[1]

Long-term retrospective studies have demonstrated durable oncologic control with PN, but, in the case of early reported series, these have been generally limited by selection bias. Fergany and colleagues[3] reported early results of patients treated with nephron-sparing surgery (NSS) with mean follow up of 104 plus or minus 57 months. The 10-year cancer-specific survival (CSS) survival rate was 73%; however, the cohort was distinct from current series in that 90% of patients

[a] Division of Urologic Oncology, New York University Langone Medical Center, 150 East 32nd Street, Suite 200, New York, NY 10016, USA
[b] Division of Urologic Oncology, Department of Urology, NYU Langone Medical Center, NYU Cancer Institute, 150 East 32nd Street, New York, NY 10016, USA
* Corresponding author.
E-mail address: samir.taneja@nyumc.org

Urol Clin N Am 39 (2012) 199–210
doi:10.1016/j.ucl.2012.02.003
0094-0143/12/$ – see front matter Published by Elsevier Inc.

underwent PN for absolute indications, and greater than one-third of patients had pT3 disease. In the subset of patients who underwent elective PN for unilateral disease and tumors less than 4 cm, the CSS and disease-free survival (DFS) rate was 100% at 10 years. Another study evaluating the survival of 70 patients undergoing PN demonstrated 10-year DFS and overall survival (OS) rates of 97% and 93%, respectively.[4] Lau and colleagues[5] also retrospectively reviewed long-term survival in a matched cohort of 164 patients with T1 tumors undergoing elective RN or PN and found no difference in 10-year OS (73% vs 74%) and CSS (98% vs 96%).

Most reported outcomes for PN have been from retrospectively evaluated series, which have the inherent potential for selection bias when comparing outcomes with RN. One randomized prospective phase 3 trial was conducted comparing open RN and PN in 541 patients with clinical tumors no more than 5 cm and a normal contralateral kidney. At a median follow up of 9.3 years, the total of number of deaths was 117, and the total number of cancer-related deaths was 12. The intention-to-treat (ITT) analysis demonstrated that the 10-year OS for patients who underwent RN was significantly better than for those undergoing PN (81.1% vs 75.7%, respectively; $P = .03$) The authors performed a secondary analysis in which they excluded patients with pathologic multifocality and upstaging. In this analysis, there was no difference in OS observed in either group. Oncologic equivalence with regard to CSS and progression could not be definitively demonstrated due to the limited number of cancer-related deaths as well as the small sample size. The authors did demonstrate similar 10-year progression rates of 4.1% and 3.3% ($P = .48$) with PN and RN, respectively. Major limitations of the study included its early termination because of poor accrual (such that the required sample size of 1300 patients was not reached) and the high rate of crossover following randomization.[6]

Local recurrence rates, defined as any disease presence in the treated kidney or associated renal fossa after treatment, are comparable between RN and PN regardless of surgical technique. Local recurrence-free survival for open RN is 98.1%, and for open PN (OPN), it is 98.0% at median follow-up 58.3 and 46.9 months, respectively. When comparing laparoscopic technique, local recurrence-free survival for RN is 99.2%, and for PN, it is 98.4% at a median follow up of 17.7 months and 15 months, respectively. It is important to note that in these studies, the median tumor size was larger in patients undergoing RN.[7]

Impact of Surgical Margins on Oncologic Outcomes

In performing a PN for tumor, the fundamental tenet of the operation has classically been complete excision with a clear margin of normal parenchyma surrounding the tissue. The significance of a positive surgical margin (PSM) has been evaluated by a number of authors.

Yossepowitch and colleagues[8] evaluated patients who underwent PN at 2 tertiary care centers with median follow-up of 3.4 years. Of the 1390 patients, 77 had PSMs. When stratified by surgical margin status, at 5 years the freedom of local recurrence was 98% and not statistically different from patients with negative surgical margins. Another multi-institutional retrospective study evaluated the natural history and the impact of PSMs on survival. Of 111 patients with PSMs with mean follow up of 37 months, 93 were monitored, while 18 patients underwent immediate reoperation with either PN or RN based upon surgeon preference. Only 40% of patients who underwent reoperation demonstrated residual tumor. Of the patients who underwent surveillance, there was no difference in CSS and OS at a mean follow-up of 37 months. On multivariate analysis, PSMs did not impact occurrence of recurrence. Given the slow growth rates described in the literature, the authors suggested that the impact of PSMs may require more years to become apparent and that median follow up of 3 years may be inadequate.[9]

The excision of the tumor with a substantial margin of normal parenchyma is considered the standard technique to reduce risk of local recurrence; however, the minimal thickness of tumor-free surgical margin has not been specified. Simple enucleation consists of incision of the renal parenchyma within a few millimeters of the tumor and blunt dissection of a plane between the capsule of the tumor and healthy renal tissue without the inclusion in the removed tissue of any visible normal renal parenchyma. One study compared oncologic outcomes of 982 patients who underwent PN with 537 patients who had simple enucleation for renal tumors with mean follow-up of 51 and 54.4 months, respectively. There was no difference in local recurrence and oncologic control, with similar CSS at 5 and 10 years. It is important to note that most patients in the enucleation group were found to have a negative margin.[10]

Despite the literature supporting the idea that no intervention is necessary for patients with a positive margin at PN, margin control remains, in the authors' opinion, a critical component of the operation. One should not conclude from this literature that the margin is not an important goal of the operation, as pathologic positive margins may in many cases be artifactual due to tissue distortion or parenchymal retraction. This concept is supported by the observation that only 40% of patients are found to have residual tumor upon completion RN.[9] Grossly positive margins, in which the surgeon violates the tumor capsule, or cuts into the tumor, would likely carry a much higher risk of local recurrence. As such, the authors continue to strive for achieving a 1 cm negative margin thickness at the time of PN to avoid inadvertently positive surgical margins.

Surgical Outcomes of Partial Nephrectomy: Complications

Although the oncologic equivalence of PN to RN for localized renal tumors has been demonstrated in the literature, patients undergoing PN are at potential increased risk for postoperative complications. The risks and benefits of PN should be addressed when counseling patients about NSS. Complications of PN include bleeding, urine leak, renal dysfunction, vascular fistula or malformation, positive margin, renal infarct, and renal loss.

A multi-institutional retrospective study by Stephenson and colleagues[11] reviewed complications associated with OPN and RN. Although patients undergoing PN did not experience more complications than those who underwent RN (19% vs 16%, $P = .3$), they did experience more grade 3 (4% vs 1.6%, $P = .04$) and procedure-related complications, defined as urinary leak, acute renal failure (ARF), retroperitoneal hemorrhage, organ injury (9% vs 3%, $P = .0001$). In the cohort of PN patients, the rate of postoperative hemorrhage requiring transfusion was 0.8%, and the rate of urinary leak was 6.6%, with a median time to fistula closure of 46 days. On multivariate analysis, patient age, operative time, and pathologic stage were associated with postoperative complications.

As experience and comfort level increased with PN, the complication rates have decreased. Thompson and colleagues reviewed their contemporary experience (1996–2001) with historical controls (1985–1995). In the contemporary cohort, there were significant decreases in the duration of hospitalization, intraoperative blood loss, and early complications (13.4% vs 6.9%, $P = .002$). Rates of urinary leakage also decreased in the contemporary group compared with the historic controls (0.6% vs 2.6%).[12]

With the introduction of minimally invasive techniques, such as laparoscopy and robotics, patients benefit with decreased postoperative pain, shorter hospital stay, and improved cosmesis.

However, the principles of PN in the open approach should be adhered to such that ischemia time and postoperative complications are minimal. A multi-institutional comparison of 1800 laparoscopic nephrectomy and OPN for solitary renal tumors evaluated the intraoperative and postoperative outcomes of these 2 techniques. The baseline characteristics were different between the groups, with more patients undergoing OPN for solitary kidneys, bilateral renal tumors, and larger renal tumors. Intraoperatively, patients who underwent laparoscopic partial nephrectomy (LPN) had 1.69 times longer warm ischemia times, more postoperative complications (18.6% vs 13.7%), including increased risk of postoperative hemorrhage (4.2% vs 1.6%), and increased risk of requiring a secondary procedure, compared with OPN.[13] It is important to note that, as in the case of OPN, complication rates with LPN are likely to have decreased with operator experience.

Theoretical advantages of the robotic technique compared with pure laparoscopy include ease of suturing during reconstruction, resulting in reduced ischemia time. A single institutional study retrospectively evaluated outcomes for minimally invasive PN (laparoscopic and robotic) with OPN for pT1b tumors. There was no difference in tumor stage, margin status, complications, or postoperative use of narcotics; however, there was statistically significant difference in ischemia time and estimated blood loss in the OPN group, with more patients requiring transfusion. These differences can be explained by more patients undergoing OPN with hypothermia at the time of renal artery clamping (allowing more prolonged ischemic interval) as well as a subset undergoing OPN without renal artery clamping. Despite the noted differences, there was no difference in renal function 6 months after surgery.[14]

None of the existing literature can account for surgeon experience and case selection when comparing PN technique with regard to risk of complications. Certain types of complication do appear to be greater within each technique, but overall complication rates have substantially declined in the contemporary era. In selecting an operative approach, one must gauge operator experience and focus upon avoidance of complications unique to the technique (ie, vascular complications with robot assisted laparoscopic partial nephrectomy (RALPN), pulmonary complications with OPN).

Renal Function Outcomes After PN

Treatment of RCC extends beyond cancer control and requires a thorough understanding of the risks of competing causes of mortality. There is growing concern regarding the management of localized renal tumors and the development of postoperative renal insufficiency, because it has been demonstrated that CKD is associated with an increased risk of cardiovascular morbidity, hospitalization, and death.[15] The relation of CKD and overall mortality is imperative when counseling patients concerning treatment options. Surgeons managing these patients should be aware of factors impacting postoperative renal function, including: preoperative renal function, ischemia time, amount of normal parenchymal excision, and comorbid conditions (ie, diabetes, atherosclerotic disease, hypertension).

Impact of preoperative renal function on postoperative renal function

It has long been accepted that patients with substantial CKD are poor candidates for RN. Individuals with severe renal dysfunction, in whom RN may result in the need for dialysis, have generally been considered to have relative, or even absolute, indications for PN. It has recently, however, been demonstrated that individuals typically considered to have an elective indication for PN may have some CKD when renal function is measured by more accurate methods than serum creatinine alone. Among all individuals presenting for resection of an early stage renal tumor, those undergoing RN have a statistically significant greater risk for CKD after surgery (hazard ratio [HR] 3.8, P<.0001).[16] A multi-institutional retrospective study demonstrated that approximately one-third of patients with an eGFR greater than 60 mL/minute/1.73 m2 will develop CKD stage 3 or greater after PN. The risk of developing CKD was independent of coexisting medical conditions such as coronary artery disease, diabetes mellitus, or hypertension.[17] Despite the lack of relationship up to 25% of patients considered to have elective indications for PN with a small kidney tumor have been found to have pre-existing CKD.[18] As such, even those with elective indications may often harbor underlying renal disease that will increase the risk of worsening renal function after PN.

The significance of long-term renal function is related to its overall risk to health. CKD and cardiovascular disease appear to act as strong independent risk factors for mortality.[19] In a study using the Surveillance, Epidemiology and End Results (SEER) cancer registry linked to Medicare claims, RN was associated with an increased number of cardiovascular events and worsened OS compared with PN in patients with pT1a tumors.[20] These findings have been supported by other studies as well. In a series from the Mayo Clinic, younger patients (<65 years) treated with RN

instead of PN for pT1a tumors had a worsened overall survival. (relative risk [RR] 2.34, 95% confidence interval [CI], 1.17–4.69, P = .016).[21] In a population-based cohort of patients from the SEER cancer registry matched for age, tumor size, and year of surgery, RN was associated with a 1.23-fold increase in overall mortality than PN (P = .001). In a competing risk analysis, RN was associated with a higher rate of noncancer-related mortality.[22]

Given the collective risk of renal dysfunction in all patients undergoing surgery, careful assessment of baseline renal function will allow better patient selection and operative planning. Better tools for assessment of renal function and relative risk of renal dysfunction are needed.

Modifiable factors: ischemia time and amount of parenchyma excised

The greatest modifiable risk factors for prevention of CKD in patients undergoing PN are the amount of parenchyma removed and the extent of ischemic injury experienced by the renal remnant. Acceptable threshold ischemia times and impact on postoperative complications and long-term renal function have been demonstrated in patients undergoing PN with solitary kidneys. Because measurement of individual renal moiety functional change remains a challenge, the most meaningful data regarding renal ischemia and its relationship with long-term renal function are typically derived from solitary kidney data.

Among the most important factors affecting immediate and long-term renal function in patients with a solitary kidney undergoing PN are ischemia time and type. A retrospective multi-institutional study evaluated the impact of ischemia time during NSS in 537 patients with solitary kidneys. All patients had OPN and were performed under warm ischemia, cold ischemia, or no ischemia. Patients with warm and cold ischemia had statistically larger tumors than patients not requiring ischemia. However, after adjusting for tumor size, patients requiring warm or cold ischemia were significantly more likely to have complications (ARF, urine leak, temporary dialysis). The odds ratio of developing ARF was 3.75 and 7.11, respectively. Although there was a significant difference in developing chronic renal insufficiency (CRI) postoperatively, there was no difference in the incidence of permanent dialysis among the 3 groups. When evaluating the subset of patients treated with warm ischemia, the authors concluded that more than 20 minutes of warm ischemia were associated with an increased risk of acute and chronic renal failure and the need for permanent dialysis. Additionally, cold ischemia of greater than 35 minutes was associated with an increased risk of ARF and urine leak, but no difference in CRI or dialysis.[23]

La Rochelle and colleagues[24] found similar threshold times for warm and cold ischemia and also observed that most patients with tumors in a solitary kidney present with evidence of CKD. With median follow-up 40 months (range 0.2–148 months), no variables, including type of ischemia or absence of ischemia, were associated with degree of decrease in late GFR values. The authors suggested that the greatest risk of developing end-stage renal disease (ESRD) was local recurrence (LR) requiring nephrectomy.

Lane and colleagues[25] investigated the functional outcomes of patients who underwent PN or RN for clinical stage T1 renal cell carcinoma to determine whether RN is comparable to PN with extended ischemia. Preoperative renal function was similar in all groups (eGFR >80 mL/min/1.73 m^2) compared including patients with limited ischemia (<30 min), extended ischemia (>30 min), and RN. At last follow-up, there were significantly more patients with postoperative eGFR <45 mL/minute/1.73 m^2 who underwent RN compared with limited and extended ischemia (35%, 6.1%, and 14%, respectively, $P<.001$). They demonstrated that although outcomes in patients with extended ischemia may be poorer than in those with more limited duration ischemia, they are better than with RN.

Cold ischemia has traditionally been used during PN based on the beneficial effects observed during kidney transplantation and other renovascular surgery necessitating prolonged ischemic intervals. Lane and colleagues assessed the outcomes following PN in a solitary kidney with multivariate analysis of modifiable and nonmodifiable factors to evaluate the determinants of renal function after PN. Among 660 patients with solitary kidneys who underwent PN, patients in whom surgery was performed with cold ischemia were older and had poorer baseline renal function. There was no difference in development of postoperative acute kidney injury in the postoperative period ($P = .4$) among those with cold ischemia as compared with those without. On multivariate analysis of early and late renal function, the strongest predictors were preoperative GFR and percentage of parenchyma preserved ($P<.00001$), while ischemia time and type were not. This study was the first to evaluate percentage of parenchyma preserved and its effects on postoperative renal function, and it draws into question some of the conventional assumptions regarding the influence of ischemia.[26]

While minimization of ischemia remains a critical goal of PN, it is clear that multiple factors, modifiable and nonmodifiable, influence long-term renal function. In planning PN, the strategy to reduce ischemia must be balanced with the desire to maximally preserve parenchyma. Given the decreased visualization during tumor excision without ischemia, for example, there may be a tendency to widen the margin, thereby removing more normal parenchyma. These relationships warrant further evaluation to determine if short ischemic intervals are preferable to no ischemia at all.

CANDIDATE SELECTION

Absolute indications for PN include tumor in a solitary kidney or bilateral tumors. Baseline azotemia whereby RN would likely result in the need for dialysis also confers an absolute indication. Relative indications for PN include pre-existing medical renal disease and medical conditions that predispose to renal disease such as diabetes, hypertension, and atherosclerotic vascular disease. Multifocal tumors associated with a genetic syndrome are also considered a relative indication for PN. The most difficult decision for the contemporary urologist is in the consideration of elective partial nephrectomy for T1a, T1b, and T2 or T3 tumors (**Table 1**).

PN for pT1a (<4 cm) Tumors

Although the use of PN for tumors under 4 cm remains poor across the United States,[27] the American Urological Association guidelines suggest that NSS should be recommended as the standard of care for T1a tumors.[2,7] Long-term studies have demonstrated equivalent 5- and 10-year CSS in these patients when managed with PN. A population-based study using the SEER database noted an increase (7.1% to 35.9%) in use of PN between 1988 and 2004 in patients with pT1a tumors. When compared with RN, there was no difference in cancer-specific mortality at 5 years.[28] Lee and colleagues[29] compared RN and PN for T1a tumors and found equivalent oncologic results a 5 years, with a disease free survival of 96% and no local recurrences. The overall rates of local recurrence following NSS in several studies range from 0% to 10%, and when considering tumors smaller than 4 cm, the incidence is 1% to 3%.[1,30,31]

PN in pT1b (4–7 cm) Tumors

Favorable outcomes with PN in early series led several surgeons to propose the use of PN in patients with pT1b tumors favorably located in the kidney. Increasing evidence of the benefit of PN with regard to renal function has supported this position. As a result, PN is becoming an emerging standard treatment for T1b tumors

Table 1
Cancer-specific survival of nephron-sparing surgery stratified by to pathologic stage

Study	Study Design	Mean/Median Follow-up (mo)	N	Surgery Type	OS (%) 5 y	OS (%) 10 y	CSS (%) 5 y	CSS (%) 10 y	LR (%)
pT1a									
Fergany et al[3,a]	Retrospective	104	117[a]	Open	—	—	97.6[a]	94.5[a]	0[a]
Crepel et al[28]	Retrospective (m)	24	1564	Open	—	—	97.4	—	—
Van Poppel et al[6,b]	Prospective (r)	111.6	268	Open	—	75.2%	—	—	2.2%
pT1b									
Crepel et al[18]	Retrospective (m)	30	275	Open	—	—	91.4	—	—
Weight et al[33]	Retrospective	49	212	Open/lap	94.5	—	97.8	86	—
pT2/T3									
Weight et al[35]	Retrospective	53	96	Open	—	—	82	—	—
Breau et al[34]	Retrospective (m)	38.4	69	Open	—	—	—	—	6

Abbreviations: CSS, cancer-specific survival; LR, local recurrence; m, matched; OS, overall survival; r, randomized.
[a] 90% of cohort underwent nephron-sparing surgery (NSS) for imperative indications, and 29 of 117 patients met criteria for elective NSS (unifocal <4 cm tumors).
[b] ≤5 cm tumors, no difference CSS between patients treated radical nephrectomy or partial nephrectomy.

provided the operation is technically feasible and the tumor can be entirely and adequately removed.[2] A population-based study that evaluated PN with RN in patients with pT1bN0M0 demonstrated equivalent cancer-specific mortality; 5141 patients in the SEER database had renal tumors between 4 and 7 cm, of whom 275 (5.4%) underwent NSS. The 5-year cancer-specific mortality rate for PN compared with RN was 91.4% versus 95.3%, respectively (P = .2).[18] Another bi-institutional study evaluated survival in patients with 4 to 7 cm renal tumors. Of the 1159 patients with pT1b tumors, 286 (25%) underwent a PN. There was no statistical difference of CSS at a median follow-up of 4.8 years.[32]

Weight and colleagues retrospectively compared the OS and CSS in patients with pT1b tumors and no history of CKD who underwent PN (n = 212; median follow-up 41 months) or RN (n = 298, median follow-up 49 months). Patients who underwent RN were more likely to have cancer on final pathology (90% vs 80%, P = .001), upstaging on final pathology (26 vs 11%, P = .0001), and higher Fuhrman grade. They demonstrated 5-year CSS of 97.8% and 95% in patients undergoing PN and RN, respectively. However, there was difference in 5-year OS between PN and RN cohort, 94.5% vs 82.6%, P<.0001, respectively. Patients undergoing RN were at increased risk of CKD by 3.4-fold in this cohort of patients who had preoperative normal renal function. On multivariate analysis, postoperative renal function and PN were both significant predictors of improved OS, even when controlling for pathologic T stage, age, and comorbid disease. The authors suggested that the improvement in OS of patients undergoing PN may be attributable to better preservation of renal function.[33] It is possible that observed differences in survival are also, in part, due to baseline differences in overall health not measured in the study.

PN in Locally Advanced Disease, pT2 (>7 cm), and pT3

Despite increasing use of PN in patients with localized tumors, the role of PN for locally advanced disease remains unclear due to an increased risk of complications, increased risk of local recurrence, and decreased efficacy in oncologic control.

Breau and colleagues[34] compared outcomes of 69 patients with unilateral advanced disease (pT2 and pT3) treated with PN to a matched cohort of 207 patients treated with RN. At a median follow-up of 3.2 years, there was no significant difference in local recurrence, metastasis, or CSS. The authors concluded that despite equivalent short-term oncologic control, the limitations of the study include short follow-up and small sample size. In addition, they noted an increased risk of complications compared with smaller tumors because of the complexity of the resection and reconstruction and recommended diligent postoperative surveillance. Another retrospective study evaluated the outcomes of patients undergoing PN or RN for cT1 tumors that were upstaged on pathology to T2 or T3 disease. When 96 patients who underwent PN were compared with the 117 patients who underwent RN for locally advanced disease, there was equivalent cancer control at median follow-up of 53 months. Multivariate analysis of CSS demonstrated that Fuhrman grade and pathologic stage predicted survival, but age, tumor size, and type of nephrectomy did not. The authors concluded that PN did not compromise oncologic outcomes.[35]

In evaluating these studies, one must make a clear distinction between patients with clinically localized tumors that are upstaged to pT3 disease and those with cT3 disease noted on initial evaluation. Since the latter are likely at greater risk of metastatic progression, the benefit of PN in this cohort is questionable. With only limited data, the concept of locoregional control in the setting of potential systemic disease requires further evaluation with regard to oncologic equivalence to RN.

Conclusions Regarding Candidate Selection

Patients with cT1a tumors should managed with nephron-sparing strategies because of the established evidence of oncologic equivalence and reduction of risk of CKD. Those with cT1b tumors should also be offered PN unless location and complexity prevent safe excision. The benefit of PN in patients with locally advanced disease is less clear, as retrospective studies evaluating oncologic outcomes in these patients typically examine a cohort of patients undergoing PN for cT1 tumors, upgraded to pT3 on pathology. These patients are distinct from those with cT2/T3 or M+ disease. As such, patients with clinically locally advanced tumors, hematuria suggestive of collecting system invasion, and known metastatic disease should be considered as candidates for PN only when an absolute indication exists. In the future, further data regarding oncologic efficacy of PN in the M-, locally advanced patient may justify an elective approach.

Given the favorable oncologic outcomes and the relative risk of CKD with RN, only the location of the tumor and complexity of the resection should seem to influence the decision for PN among early stage tumors. As such, surgeons should gauge their own surgical outcomes and comfort level using standardized parameters such as R.E.N.A.L. (renal, exophytic/endophytic, nearness to collecting system or sinus, anterior/posterior/location relative to polar lines). nephrometry score (**Fig. 1**) to assess outcomes,[36] and consider referral of complex lesions to more experienced surgeons given the importance of nephron sparing in this group.

SURGICAL APPROACH

Surgical technique employed is surgeon dependent. With increasing experience with minimally invasive techniques, complication rates are comparable to open PN with the benefit of decreased postoperative pain and shorter hospital stay (**Table 2**). This was affirmed by a multi-institutional comparison of 1800 LPNs and OPNs for solitary renal tumors evaluated the intraoperative and postoperative outcomes of these 2 techniques. The laparoscopic technique was associated with shorter operative time, shorter hospital stays, and less intra-operative blood loss although transfusion rates were not statistically different.[13] Although in this series patients undergoing LPN had more postoperative complications, it is important to note that complication rates were relatively high, perhaps due to inclusion of the early learning curve with LPN.

Spana and colleagues[37] evaluated the complications in 450 patients who underwent robotic PN at 4 high volume centers. Mean tumor size was 2.9 cm. The rate of postoperative transfusion and interventional embolization was 3% and 1%, respectively, and was comparable to the published bleeding complications rate (0.8%).[11] In their series, venous thromboembolism (VTE) prophylaxis consisted of intermittent pneumatic compression without routine pharmacologic prophylaxis, and VTE incidence rates were similar after open and laparoscopic partial or radical nephrectomy. The rate of urinary fistula was 1.6% and was similar to contemporary open series (0.6%).[12] A limitation of the study included no objective renal scoring system to characterize complexity of tumors resected. Larger studies evaluating a matched cohort of patients with regard to preoperative variables and tumor size and complexity are needed to reliably compare outcomes these different techniques.

Complex scenarios for PN such as centrally located tumor, tumor in a solitary kidney, predominantly cystic tumor, and multifocal disease probably are best managed with an open technique in most surgeons' hands. These challenging situations, have, however, been successfully addressed by experienced minimally invasive surgeons.[38–40] Clearly, the short-term morbidity of any technique is directly related to operator experience and technical skill in the procedure. As such, comparative studies of complication rates in single institutions are subject to considerable bias, depending upon

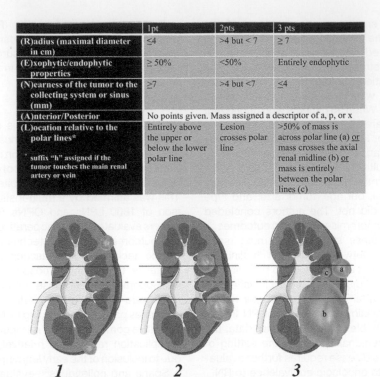

	1pt	2pts	3 pts
(R)adius (maximal diameter in cm)	≤4	>4 but < 7	≥ 7
(E)xophytic/endophytic properties	≥ 50%	<50%	Entirely endophytic
(N)earness of the tumor to the collecting system or sinus (mm)	≥7	>4 but <7	≤4
(A)nterior/Posterior	No points given. Mass assigned a descriptor of a, p, or x		
(L)ocation relative to the polar lines* * suffix "h" assigned if the tumor touches the main renal artery or vein	Entirely above the upper or below the lower polar line	Lesion crosses polar line	>50% of mass is across polar line (a) or mass crosses the axial renal midline (b) or mass is entirely between the polar lines (c)

Fig. 1. R.E.N.A.L. Nephrometry Score with scoring of (L)ocation component. Polar lines (*solid lines*) and axial renal midline (*broken line*) are depicted on each sagittal view of kidney. Numbers 1 to 3 represent points attributed to each category of tumor. (*Data from* Thompson RH, Boorjian SA, Lohse CM, et al. Radical nephrectomy for pT1a renal masses may be associated with decreased overall survival compared with partial nephrectomy. J Urol 2008;179(2):468–71; and *From* Kutikov A, Uzzo RG. The R.E.N.A.L. nephrtomy score: a comprehensive standardized system for quantitating renal tumor size, location, and depth. J Urol 2009;183:846; with permission.)

the experience of the institution. Ultimately, the decision to perform an open, laparoscopic, or robotic PN depends on the surgical experience and comfort. The contemporary literature does not convincingly support 1 technique over another, but does illustrate the strengths of each approach: the ability to cool the kidney, prolong ischemia, and, perhaps, deal more easily with complex lesions using an open approach; less pain and shorter length of stay with minimally invasive approaches. To date, there is no convincing evidence that robotic PN offers great advantage over LPN in the hands of expert operators, but the easier learning curve and the evolving experience leave this open for future evaluation.

Regardless of technique that is employed during PN, there is a growing body of literature regarding the effect of renal ischemia on short- and long-term renal function. It is clear that long-term renal function is better preserved by PN than RN, and that long-term decline in renal function influences the patient's overall health and longevity. Methods of better preserving renal function at the time of PN are less well-delineated. Most importantly, baseline renal function, risk factors for CKD, and

amount of renal parenchyma removed all strongly influence the final outcome in renal function. It is clear that many other factors, besides renal ischemic interval, affect the impact of ischemia on renal function. The long-standing belief that cold ischemia is better than warm, and the new belief that every minute counts, remain to be validated. It is likely that there is no fixed safe threshold for ischemia time, but rather it is dependent on the patient's age, comorbidities and preexisting renal function. However, ischemia time is a modifiable factor that is in part surgeon dependent, and techniques have been proposed to minimize or eliminate ischemia.

Partial Ischemia or Segmental Arterial Occlusion

With increased experience and comfort level with minimally invasive approaches, advances have been made in minimizing ischemia, which has been demonstrated in the open technique. Ukimura and colleagues[41] have suggested that 3-dimensional reconstruction of the renovascular tumor anatomy allows precise anatomy-based surgical

Table 2
Outcome of open, laparoscopic and robotic partial nephrectomy

	Surgery Type	N	Mean/Median Tumor Size (cm)	Ischemia Time (min)	PSMs	EBL (mL)	Transfusion Rate (%)	LOS (d)	Urine Leak (%)	Postoperative Hemorrhage (%)
Thompson et al[12]	OPN	480	3.0	12(w) & 27(c)	—	483	—	5.7	0.6	1.2
Gill et al[13]	OPN	1028	3.5	20.1(w)	1.3	376	5.1	5.8	2.3	1.6
	LPN	771	2.7	30.7(w)	2.9	300	4.5	3.3	3.1	4.2
Spana et al[37]	RPN	450	2.9	20.2(w)	—	206	4.0	—	1.6	—
Petros et al[46]	RPN	362	2.3	17(w)	—	150	3	2.5	0.83	1.4
	RPN	83	5	24(w)	—	200	12	3	2.4	1.2

Abbreviations: c, cold ischemia; EBL, estimated blood loss; LOS, length of stay; LPN, laparoscopic partial nephrectomy; OPN, open partial nephrectomy; PSMs, positive surgical margins; RPN, robotic partial nephrectomy; w, warm ischemia.

planning for targeted vascular microdissection to facilitate zero-ischemia PN, even for intrarenal or central tumors.[42] Gill and colleagues[43] further described their results in 58 patients who underwent zero-ischemia laparoscopic or robotic PN. Although 1 patient required hilar clamping, the remaining 57 patients had transient clamping of tertiary or higher-order arterial branches. There were no intraoperative complications and minimal postoperative complications, including urine leak (5.3%) but no postoperative hemorrhage despite 19% patients requiring transfusions. In a subset of patients who were evaluated with mercapto acetyl triglycine (MAG-3) scans, the decrease in renal function corresponded to mean percent kidney that was excised. The authors suggest their low rates of delayed post-operative hemorrhage could be attributed to the unclamped hilum during surgery, which allowed bleeding during tumor excision to be immediately evident and repaired. Partial clamping of the renal artery (<50% of arterial diameter is occluded) has also been described in the literature.[44] It is likely that targeted segmental arterial occlusion will be favored in the future; however, the feasibility, reproducibility and long-term benefits compared with traditional PN need to be established.

Nonclamped PN

Clamping of the renal pedicle is often used during PN to maintain hemostasis and adequate visualization of the surgical bed for complete tumor resection. An advantage of OPN is the potential ability to perform surgery without vascular clamping with little compromise of exposure and resection. Thompson and colleagues[23] evaluated the renal effect of vascular clamping in 537 patients with solitary kidneys undergoing PN. They found that both warm and cold ischemia were associated with an increased risk of urine leak, renal failure, and temporary dialysis; however, significantly fewer patients required temporary dialysis and developed CRI when PN was performed without vascular clamping.

The Lahey Clinic described their experience of PN in the absence of vascular clamping in 190 patients. When compared with 116 patients who underwent clamped PN, patients who underwent PN without pedicle clamping had larger tumors but no difference in PSMs, recurrence rates, or overall complications despite a greater rate of postoperative urine leak. In the subset of patients with solitary kidneys, there was a statistically significant difference in eGFR with a greater percentage decrease in patients undergoing PN with renal pedicle clamping (21% vs 4.4%, $P =$ .027).[45] While continued efforts are ongoing to evolve techniques of clampless PN, it is important to note that these are advanced techniques with increased risk of morbidity in inexperienced hands. The major priority for surgeons should be adaptation of PN, and techniques such as these should be adopted once the surgeon feels truly facile with the traditional operation.

SUMMARY

PN has become the preferred surgical technique for early stage localized renal tumors. The oncologic efficacy of PN in pT1a tumors has been demonstrated in the literature, and there is a growing body of evidence suggesting equivalent oncologic control in pT1b tumors. The oncologic efficacy and the growing evidence to suggest harm from RN have swayed the pendulum strongly to the side of nephron sparing. When considering patients for surgical treatment, an attempt should be made to perform NSS in nearly all patients with T1a lesions, and in most patients with T1b lesions reasonably located within the kidney. While PN can be considered among individuals with locally advanced disease, there is insufficient evidence, to date, to suggest it as a routine. As there is no clear evidence favoring 1 approach over others, the selection of a surgical approach for PN should be dependent upon surgeon experience. The goals of resection should be complete excision with negative margins, minimized renal ischemia, and as minimal renal parenchymal resection as necessary to achieve complete tumor excision.

REFERENCES

1. Nguyen CT, Campbell SC, Novick AC. Choice of operation for clinically localized renal tumor. Urol Clin North Am 2008;35(4):645–55.
2. Van Poppel H, Becker F, Cadeddu JA, et al. Treatment of localized renal cell carcinoma. Eur Urol 2011;60(4):662–72.
3. Fergany AF, Hafez KS, Novick AC. Long-term results of nephron sparing surgery for localized renal cell carcinoma: 10-year followup. J Urol 2000;163(2):442–5.
4. Herr HW. Partial nephrectomy for unilateral renal carcinoma and a normal contralateral kidney: 10-year followup. J Urol 1999;161(1):33–4 [discussion: 34–5].
5. Lau WK, Blute ML, Weaver AL, et al. Matched comparison of radical nephrectomy vs nephron-sparing surgery in patients with unilateral renal cell carcinoma and a normal contralateral kidney. Mayo Clin Proc 2000;75(12):1236–42.

6. Van Poppel H, Da Pozzo L, Albrecht W, et al. A prospective, randomised EORTC intergroup phase 3 study comparing the oncologic outcome of elective nephron-sparing surgery and radical nephrectomy for low-stage renal cell carcinoma. Eur Urol 2011;59(4):543–52.

7. Novick AC, Campbell SC, Belldegrun A, et al. AUA guidelines 2009: guideline for management of the clinical stage 1 renal mass. J Urol 2009;182(4):1271–9.

8. Yossepowitch O, Thompson RH, Leibovich BC, et al. Positive surgical margins at partial nephrectomy: predictors and oncological outcomes. J Urol 2008; 179(6):2158–63.

9. Bensalah K, Pantuck AJ, Rioux-Leclercq N, et al. Positive surgical margin appears to have negligible impact on survival of renal cell carcinomas treated by nephron-sparing surgery. Eur Urol 2010;57(3): 466–71.

10. Minervini A, Ficarra V, Rocco F, et al. Simple enucleation is equivalent to traditional partial nephrectomy for renal cell carcinoma: results of a nonrandomized, retrospective, comparative study. J Urol 2011; 185(5):1604–10.

11. Stephenson AJ, Hakimi AA, Snyder ME, et al. Complications of radical and partial nephrectomy in a large contemporary cohort. J Urol 2004;171(1):130–4.

12. Thompson RH, Leibovich BD, Lohse CM, et al. Complications of contemporary open nephron sparing surgery: a single institution experience. J Urol 2005;174(3):855–8.

13. Gill IS, Kavoussi LR, Lane BR, et al. Comparison of 1,800 laparoscopic and open partial nephrectomies for single renal tumors. J Urol 2007;178(1):41–6.

14. Sprenkle PC, Power N, Ghoneim T, et al. Comparison of open and minimally invasive partial nephrectomy for renal tumors 4-8 centimeters. Eur Urol 2012; 61(3):593–9.

15. Go AS, Chertow GM, Fan D, et al. Chronic kidney disease and the risks of death, cardiovascular events, and hospitalization. N Engl J Med 2004; 351(13):1296–305.

16. Huang WC, Levey AS, Serio AM, et al. Chronic kidney disease after nephrectomy in patients with renal cortical tumors: a retrospective cohort study. Lancet Oncol 2006;7(9):735–40.

17. Clark MA, Shikanov S, Raman JD, et al. Chronic kidney disease before and after partial nephrectomy. J Urol 2011;185(1):43–8.

18. Crepel M, Jeldres C, Peorrotte P, et al. Nephron-sparing surgery is equally effective for radical nephrectomy for T1BN0M0 renal cell carcinoma: a population-based assessment. Urology 2010;75(2):271–5.

19. Huang WC, Elkin EB, Levey AS, et al. Partial nephrectomy versus radical nephrectomy in patients with small renal tumors—is there a difference in mortality and cardiovascular outcomes? J Urol 2009;181(1):55–61.

20. Weiner DE, Tighiouart H, Stark PC, et al. Kidney disease as a risk factor for recurrent cardiovascular disease and mortality. Am J Kidney Dis 2004;44(2): 198–206.

21. Thompson RH, Boorjian SA, Lohse CM, et al. Radical nephrectomy for pT1a renal masses may be associated with decreased overall survival compared with partial nephrectomy. J Urol 2008; 179(2):468–71.

22. Zini L, Perrotte P, Capitanio U, et al. Radical versus partial nephrectomy: effect on overall and non-cancer mortality. Cancer 2009;115(7):1465–71.

23. Thompson RH, Frank I, Lohse CM, et al. The impact of ischemia time during open nephron sparing surgery on solitary kidneys: a multi-institutional study. J Urol 2007;177(2):471–6.

24. La Rochelle J, Shuch B, Riggs S, et al. Functional and oncological outcomes of partial nephrectomy of solitary kidneys. J Urol 2009;181(5):2037–42.

25. Lane BR, Fergany AF, Weight CJ, et al. Renal functional outcomes after partial nephrectomy with extended ischemic intervals are better than after radical nephrectomy. J Urol 2010;184(4):1286–90.

26. Lane BR, Russo P, Uzzo RG, et al. Comparison of cold and warm ischemia during partial nephrectomy in 660 solitary kidneys reveals predominant role of nonmodifiable factors in deteriming ultimate renal function. J Urol 2011;185(2):421–7.

27. Dulabon LM, Lowrance WT, Russo P, et al. Trends in renal tumor surgery delivery within the United States. Cancer 2010;116(10):2316–21.

28. Crepel M, Jeldres C, Sun M, et al. A population-based comparison of cancer-control rates between radical and partial nephrectomy for T1a renal cell carcinoma. Urology 2010;76(4):883–8.

29. Lee CT, Katz J, Shi W, et al. Surgical management of renal tumors 4 cm or less in a contemporary cohort. J Urol 2000;163(3):730–6.

30. Uzzo RG, Novick AC. Nephron sparing surgery for renal tumors: indications, techniques and outcomes. J Urol 2001;166(1):6–18.

31. Belldegrun A, Tsui KH, deKernion JB. Efficacy of nephron-sparing surgery for renal cell carcinoma: analysis based on the new 1997 tumor-node-metastasis staging system. J Clin Oncol 1999;17(9):2868–75.

32. Thompson RH, Siddiqui S, Lohse CM, et al. Partial versus radical nephrectomy for 4 to 7 cm renal cortical tumors. J Urol 2009;182(6):2601–6.

33. Weight CJ, Larson BT, Gao T, et al. Elective partial nephrectomy in patients with clinical T1b renal tumors is associated with improved overall survival. Urology 2010;76(3):631–7.

34. Breau RH, Crispen PL, Jimenez RE, et al. Outcome of stage T2 or greater renal cell cancer treated with partial nephrectomy. J Urol 2010;183(3):903–8.

35. Weight CJ, Lythgoe C, unnikrishnan R, et al. Partial nephrectomy does not compromise survival in

patients with pathologic upstaging to pT2/pT3 or high-grade renal tumors compared with radical nephrectomy. Urology 2011;77(5):1142–6.

36. Kutikov A, Uzzo RG. The R.E.N.A.L. nehrometry score: a comprehensive standardized system for quantitating renal tumor size, location and depth. J Urol 2009;183:844–53.

37. Spana G, Haber GP, Dulabon LM, et al. Complications after robotic partial nephrectomy at centers of excellence: multi-institutional analysis of 450 cases. J Urol 2011;186(2):417–21.

38. Gill IS, Colombo JR Jr, Frank I, et al. Laparoscopic partial nephrectomy for hilar tumors. J Urol 2005; 174(3):850–3.

39. Frank I, Colombo JR Jr, Rubinstein M, et al. Laparoscopic partial nephrectomy for centrally located renal tumors. J Urol 2006;175(3 Pt 1): 849–52.

40. Dulabon LM, Kaouk JH, Haber GP, et al. Multi-institutional analysis of robotic partial nephrectomy for hilar versus nonhilar lesions in 446 consecutive cases. Eur Urol 2011;59(3):325–30.

41. Ukimura O, Nakamoto M, Gill IS. Three-dimensional reconstruction of renovascular-tumor anatomy to facilitate zero-ischemia partial nephrectomy. Eur Urol 2012;61(1):211–7.

42. Abreu AL, Gill IS, Desai MM. Zero-ischemia robotic partial nephrectomy (RPN) for hilar tumours. BJU Int 2011;108(6 Pt 2):948–54.

43. Gill IS, Patil MB, de Castro Abreu AL, et al. Zero ischemia anatomical partial nephrectomy: a novel approach. J Urol 2012;187(3):807–15.

44. Kowalczyk KJ, Alemozaffar M, Hevelone ND, et al. Partial clamping of the renal artery during robotic-assisted laparoscopic partial nephrectomy: technique and initial outcomes. J Endourol 2012. [Epub ahead of print].

45. Smith GL, Kenney PA, Lee Y. Non-clamped partial nephrectomy: techniques and surgical outcomes. BJU Int 2011;107(7):1054–8.

46. Petros F, Sukumar S, Haber GP, et al. Multi-institutional analysis of robotic partial nephrectomy for renal tumors >4cm vs. ≤4cm in 445 consecutive patients. J Endourol 2012. [Epub ahead of print].

Integration of Surgery and Systemic Therapy for Renal Cell Carcinoma

Patrick A. Kenney, MD[a], Christopher G. Wood, MD[b],*

KEYWORDS

- Renal cell carcinoma • Adjuvant therapy
- Neoadjuvant therapy • Cytoreductive nephrectomy
- Immunotherapy • Targeted therapy • Angiogenesis inhibitor
- Tyrosine kinase inhibitor

An estimated 58,240 people in the United States were diagnosed with kidney cancer in 2010, and 13,040 died of the disease.[1] Forty percent of patients have regionally advanced or metastatic disease at diagnosis, and 10% to 28% develop recurrence or metastasis after surgery for localized disease.[1] To maximize clinical outcomes, proper integration of surgery and systemic therapy is essential. This review focuses on the role of adjuvant therapy for renal cell carcinoma (RCC), neoadjuvant therapy for locally advanced disease, and multimodal therapy for metastatic RCC (mRCC), including cytoreductive nephrectomy and presurgical targeted therapy.

NOMENCLATURE

The nomenclature of integrated systemic and surgical therapy is not standardized. For clarity, and as described in a recent collaborative review, the term adjuvant therapy is used in this review to describe treatment that is administered after complete surgical resection with the goal of reducing risk of recurrence in a patient without evidence of disease.[2] Neoadjuvant therapy refers to use of a therapy before surgical resection of clinically localized disease. Presurgical therapy designates the administration of a therapy before planned cytoreductive surgery in mRCC.

ADJUVANT THERAPY FOR RCC AT INCREASED RISK OF RELAPSE

Despite the increase in early detection in the modern era, 10% to 28% of patients develop recurrence or distant metastasis after nephrectomy for clinically localized disease.[3] Cure is elusive for patients with distant metastatic disease, with 5-year survival rates of approximately 10%.[1] A wide range of adjuvant therapies have been investigated to reduce risk of recurrence. An ideal adjuvant therapy has a favorable toxicity profile, proven activity in metastatic disease, proven efficacy against the standard of care (observation) in phase 3 randomized trials, and can be administered on an outpatient basis to patients who are most likely to benefit from adjuvant therapy.[4,5] Although no agents have reliably met these goals and observation remains the standard of care, trials of several promising therapies are in progress.

Disclosures: None (P.A.K.).
Disclosures: Pfizer (Investigator, Consultant, Speaker's Bureau); Argos (Investigator, Consultant); GlaxoSmithKline (Investigator); Bayer (Investigator); Novartis (Investigator); Wilex (Investigator) (C.G.W.).
[a] Urologic Oncology, Department of Urology, MD Anderson Cancer Center, 1515 Holcombe Boulevard, Unit 1373, Houston, TX 77030, USA
[b] Department of Urology, MD Anderson Cancer Center, 1515 Holcombe, Unit 1373, Houston, TX 77030, USA
* Corresponding author.
E-mail address: cgwood@mdanderson.org

Defining Risk of Recurrence

A recognized disadvantage of the adjuvant approach is that some patients who have been cured with surgery alone are unnecessarily treated with adjuvant systemic therapy. An essential component of developing effective adjuvant therapy is to identify the population of patients who are at high risk of recurrence and thus most likely to benefit from adjuvant therapy.

Models incorporating clinical and pathologic data

Several prognostic models have been developed that predict the risk of progression after surgery for localized RCC using clinical and pathologic variables (**Table 1**).[6–9] These models, some of which have been externally validated, may prove to be useful for selecting patients for adjuvant therapy.[5] Each model has limitations. For instance, Kattan and colleagues acknowledged that predicting 5-year recurrence-free survival limits the usefulness of their nomograms, because it does not capture the 15% to 19% rate of recurrence beyond 5 years.[3,6,10,11] In addition, the 2001 Memorial Sloan-Kettering Cancer Center (MSKCC) nomogram included both clear cell and nonclear cell histology. The investigators thus chose to exclude nuclear grade from their nomogram because of controversy regarding the grading of nonclear cell tumors.[6] Given the association between grade and outcome, the impact of excluding nuclear grade on the predictive capacity of the nomogram has been questioned.[3,6,8] The 2005 MSKCC nomogram addresses this concern by limiting the model to clear cell RCC (ccRCC), which allowed nuclear grade to be included as a predictive variable.[7]

The modified University of California at Los Angeles (UCLA) Integrated Staging System (UISS) has been externally validated.[12] Like the MSKCC nomograms, the UISS timeframe is limited to 5 years. A limitation of the UISS is that it assigns patients to low-risk, medium-risk, or high-risk groups rather than predicting risk for an individual patient.[9,13] A range of outcomes is expected within each risk category. The discriminating abilities of the 2001 MSKCC nomogram and the UISS were compared using a multicenter European cohort of 2404 patients.[14] The concordance indices were 0.71 and 0.68 for the MSKCC and UISS models, respectively. The MSKCC nomogram improved discrimination of the UISS intermediate-risk category.[14]

Additional predictive models exist that are based solely on preoperative variables such as gender, symptoms, and imaging findings,

including necrosis, lymphadenopathy, and tumor size.[15–17] The postoperative models, which include pathologic variables, discriminate better than preoperative models and are therefore more appropriate for selection of candidates for adjuvant therapy.[13,14] Nonetheless, preoperative-only models may help select intervention versus active surveillance, and may prove useful for identifying patients for neoadjuvant therapy.[13,18]

Models integrating molecular markers with clinical and pathologic data

Future efforts to determine risk of recurrence after nephrectomy may incorporate molecular markers.[5] For example, addition of data regarding expression of 3 molecular markers (carbonic anhydrase IX [CA IX], vimentin, and p53) to clinical markers (metastasis, T stage, performance status) yielded modestly improved accuracy in predicting disease-specific survival in localized and metastatic ccRCC compared with the UISS (concordance indices 0.79 vs 0.75).[19] More recently, the same group published a nomogram combining clinical, pathologic, and molecular data to predict disease-free survival after nephrectomy for localized ccRCC (**Fig. 1**).[20] The nomogram variables include expression of Ki-67, p53, endothelial vascular endothelial growth factor receptor 1 (VEGFR-1), epithelial VEGFR-1, and epithelial VEGF-D along with T stage and performance status. The predictive ability of the 5 molecular markers alone exceeded that of the UISS (concordance index 0.84 vs 0.78). The accuracy of the nomogram incorporating the clinical, pathologic, and molecular data was higher still (concordance index 0.90).

Similarly, the group from Mayo Clinic used immunohistochemistry to characterize expression of B7-H1, survivin, and Ki-67 in 634 patients treated with radical or partial nephrectomy for localized or metastatic ccRCC.[21] The 3 molecular markers were each shown to be independently associated with RCC-specific death. Weighted scores were assigned to marker expression, which was dichotomized. The total score (range 0–7), termed BioScore, was able to discriminate cancer-specific survival (**Fig. 2**). The investigators showed that the addition of BioScore improved the predictive ability of other models including TNM staging (concordance index 0.82 vs 0.79) and the UISS (0.82 vs 0.77).[21]

Predictive models that include biomarkers are promising and may help select patients for adjuvant therapy. These models require independent validation and standardization of laboratory techniques before incorporation into clinical practice.[22] Moreover, the costs of using biomarkers must be

Table 1
Models predicting the risk of progression or progression after surgery for localized RCC using clinical and pathologic variables

Author	Year	Institution	Type	Study Population (n)	Inclusion				Variables									Outcome	Timepoint (y)	Concordance Index
					TNM	Histology	Nephrectomy	Years	Symptoms	Performance Status	Tumor Size	pT	pN	Grade	Histology	Necrosis	Vascular Invasion			
Kattan et al[6]	2001	MSKCC	Nomogram	601	T1–3c, N0/x, M0	Papillary, chromophobe, ccRCC	Partial, radical	1989–1998	✓		✓	✓ (1997)		✓				Recurrence-free survival[a]	5	0.74
Zisman[9]	2002	UCLA	Algorithm (low, moderate, high risk)	468	T1–4, N0, M0	Any	Partial, radical	1989–2000		✓		✓ (1997)	✓	✓				Overall survival, disease-specific survival, local recurrence-free survival, and systemic recurrence-free survival	1, 2, 3, 4, 5	NA
Leibovich et al[8]	2003	Mayo	Algorithm (score between 0 and 11)	1671	T1–4, Nx –N2, M0	ccRCC	Radical	1970–2000			✓	✓ (2002)	✓	NA		✓	✓	Metastasis-free survival	1, 3, 5, 7, 10	0.82
Sorbellini et al[7]	2005	MSKCC	Nomogram	701	T1–3c, N0/x, M0	ccRCC	Partial, radical	1989–2002			✓	✓ (2002)	✓	NA		✓	✓	Recurrence-free survival[a]	5	0.82

Abbreviations: NA, not applicable; pN, pathologic node stage; pT, pathologic tumor stage.

[a] Local, distant or contralateral kidney recurrence.

Data from Refs.[6–9]

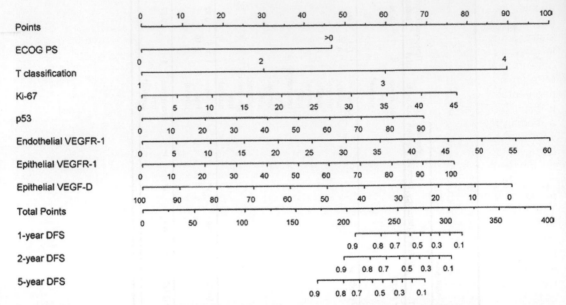

Fig. 1. Nomogram predicting disease-free survival using clinical, pathologic, and molecular data. To read the nomogram, determine the number of points assigned to each factor by drawing a vertical line to the points axis. The sum of the points corresponds to probability of disease-free survival. (*Reprinted from* Klatte T, Seligson DB, LaRochelle J, et al. Molecular signatures of localized clear cell renal cell carcinoma to predict disease-free survival after nephrectomy. Cancer Epidemiol Biomarkers Prev 2009;18:897; with permission.)

considered in context of the thus far modest improvement over the user-friendly, readily available clinicopathologic models.[3]

Reported Adjuvant Trials

Radiotherapy

Initial adjuvant studies focused on improving local control with radiotherapy.[5] Radical nephrectomy provides excellent local cancer control and

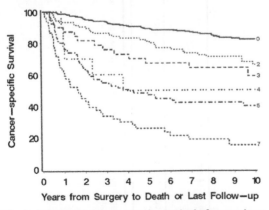

Fig. 2. Estimated cancer-specific survival after nephrectomy is discriminated by BioScore in 634 patients with ccRCC. (*Reprinted from* Parker AS, Leibovich BC, Lohse CM, et al. Development and evaluation of Bio-Score: a biomarker panel to enhance prognostic algorithms for clear cell renal cell carcinoma. Cancer 2009;115:2097; with permission.)

recurrence of RCC is typically distant from the primary. Because local failure is uncommon, little role is expected for adjuvant radiotherapy.[23] The data support this expectation.

In a prospective trial conducted from 1961 to 1970 at Newcastle General Hospital (Newcastle Upon Tyne, UK), patients with a completely resected primary tumor and no evidence of metastatic disease were randomized to observation (n = 49) or adjuvant radiation to the renal bed, incision, and para-aortic nodes (n = 51).[24] There was no significant difference in local recurrence, development of metastases, or survival. Significant side effects, including 4 deaths from liver failure, were attributed to the radiation.

In 1987, Kjaer and Frederiksen[25] reported the results of a multicenter randomized trial in Copenhagen, Denmark. Between 1979 and 1984, patients with stage II and III RCC were randomized after nephrectomy to 50 Gy of external beam radiotherapy in 20 fractions to the kidney bed and nodes (n = 32) or observation (n = 33). Radiotherapy was associated with hepatic, gastric, and duodenal injury, but no improvement in relapse. In 19% of patients, radiotherapy complications contributed to the patient's death.

Hormonal therapy

Some renal tumor cells express glucocorticoid receptors that can be blocked by hormonal agents, such as medroxyprogesterone acetate (MPA), which have reported activity in the metastatic setting.[26] In 1987, Pizzocaro and colleagues[27] reported a multicenter trial in which patients were randomized to 1 year of adjuvant MPA (n = 58) or observation (n = 62) after radical nephrectomy for nonmetastatic RCC. Sixty-two (51%) of the patients had at least T3 disease. After a median follow-up of 5 years, rates of relapse were similar in the intervention and control groups (32.7 vs 33.9%). Complications were common in the intervention group.

Immunotherapy

There is a strong rationale for immunotherapy in RCC. The essential role played by the host immune system is shown by case reports of spontaneous regression of metastatic disease after nephrectomy or ablation of the primary tumor, as well as the presence of tumor-infiltrating immune cells in nephrectomy specimens, which have shown antitumor activity.[28–32] The primary tumor is believed to have an immunosuppressive effect that can be ameliorated by nephrectomy.[33–36] The aim of immunotherapy is to augment the host immune response. Once the immune sink has been excised, it is posited that adjuvant immunotherapy can better treat the remaining subclinical disease that leads to recurrence. Various methodologies have been used, including administration of cytokines, vaccines, dendritic cell therapy, and allogeneic hematopoietic stem-cell transplant to take advantage of graft-versus-tumor effect.[37–39]

An aspect of the antitumor immune response is believed to be mediated by CD8+ cytotoxic T lymphocytes and amplified by CD4+ helper T cells, which secrete cytokines including interleukin 2 (IL-2) and interferon α (IFN-α).[22] Exogenous IL-2 and IFN-α have shown efficacy in metastatic disease, with response rates up to 20% and a 5% durable complete response for IL-2.[38,40–42] Based on these findings, several randomized trials investigated IL-2 and IFN-α as adjuvant therapy but were unable to show a disease-free or overall survival benefit (**Table 2**).[43–46] In 1 trial, adjuvant chemoimmunotherapy was associated with worse 5-year overall survival when compared with control (58 vs 76%, P = .028).[46]

Adjuvant active specific immunotherapy with vaccines has also been used, with mostly unfavorable results. In 1996, Galligioni and colleagues[47] reported a trial in which patients after nephrectomy were randomized to observation (n = 60) versus intradermal injection of irradiated tumor cells and Bacille Calmette-Guérin (n = 60). One month after completing therapy, a delayed-type

cutaneous hypersensitivity reaction to autologous tumor cells was shown in 70% of immunized patients. Despite this induced tumor-specific immunoreactivity, 5-year disease-free survival was similar in the intervention and control arms (63 vs 72%, P = nonsignificant).

In 2004, Jocham and colleagues[48] reported the only successful adjuvant trial in RCC to date. In 1997 to 1998 at 55 centers in Germany, 558 patients scheduled for radical nephrectomy were enrolled. Patients were randomized before nephrectomy to receive 6 adjuvant intradermal injections of autologous tumor vaccine at 4-week intervals or observation. After nephrectomy, only patients with pT2 to 3b, pN0 to 3, M0 RCC and Eastern Cooperative Oncology Group (ECOG) performance status 0 to 2 were permitted to continue in the trial. Patients with pT1 or pT4 disease were excluded. Tumor cells were devitalized by rapid freezing at −82°C and thawing. The primary end point was tumor progression.

Five patients withdrew consent before surgery. After surgery, 174 patients were withdrawn from the study for various reasons such as non-RCC histology, incorrect tumor stage, and inability to prepare the vaccine. More of these patients were in the vaccine arm (n = 99 vs 75). Among the remaining 379 patients, 5-year progression-free survival was higher in the vaccine group (77.4 vs 67.8%, P = .02). At 5 years, the hazard ratio for progression was 1.58 (95% confidence interval [CI] 1.05–2.37, P = .02) in favor of vaccination. The 5-year progression-free survival benefit favoring vaccination was pronounced in patients with pT3 disease (67.5 vs 49.7%, P = .039). Twelve adverse events of mild to moderate severity were reported in the vaccine group.

The trial was criticized for the large loss of patients (32%) after randomization, which was imbalanced between study arms.[49] Given the study design, in which patients were randomized before pathologic diagnosis and staging, some loss of patients was inevitable. A secondary intention-to-treat analysis was subsequently reported in abstract form with a larger number of patients in the vaccine (n = 233) and control (n = 244) groups.[50] The vaccine was still associated with improved progression-free survival (P = .048). The magnitude of the benefit was not reported. There was no difference in overall survival (P = .12). A retrospective matched-pair analysis of the same vaccine protocol in 495 patients was recently reported.[51] With median follow-up of 131 months, the tumor cell vaccine was an independent predictor of overall survival on multivariable analysis in the whole group (hazard ratio [HR] 1.28, P = .030), as well as in

Table 2
Randomized trials investigating IL-2 and IFN-α as adjuvant therapy. None showed a disease-free or overall survival benefit

First Author	Year	Eligibility	Intervention	Control	N	Median Follow-up	Primary End Point	Outcome (Intervention vs Control)	P Value
Pizzocaro et al[44]	2001	Robson II or III	IFN-α	Observation	247	NA	5-year OS	66.5% vs 66.0%	.861
Messing et al[43]	2003	pT3–4a or N+	IFN-α	Observation	283	10.4 years	Median OS	5.1 vs 7.4 years	.09
Clark et al[45]	2003	pT3b–4 or N+ or M1 (resected)	High-dose IL-2	Observation	69	22 months	2-year DFS	48% vs 55%	.431
Atzpodien et al[46]	2005	pT3b–4 or N+ or M1 (resected)	IFN-α + IL-2 + 5-fluorouracil	Observation	203	4.3 years	5-year OS	58% vs 76%	.028

Abbreviations: OS, overall surviva; pT, pathologic tumor stage.
Data from Refs.[43–46]

the subset of patients with pT3 disease (HR 1.67, $P = .011$). Despite the progression-free survival benefit noted in a randomized trial and strong corroborating retrospective evidence, the therapy was not accepted broadly into practice, which led to the insolvency of the manufacturer of the vaccine.[49]

In the largest phase 3 adjuvant trial in RCC, patients were randomized to receive vitespen (Oncophage) (n = 409) or observation (n = 409) after nephrectomy.[52] Vitespen is a heat shock protein (HSP) vaccine. HSPs are intracellular chaperones that play a role in the loading of antigenic peptides onto major histocompatibility complex class I molecules, eliciting an immune response.[5,26] Autologous HSP vaccines consist of HSP-peptide complexes, which are isolated from a patient's tumor. In an intention-to treat analysis, the rate of recurrence was similar in the vitespen and control groups (37.7 vs 39.8%, $P = .506$) after a median follow-up of 1.9 years.

Other

Thalidomide, an antiangiogenic and immunomodulatory drug, has activity in mRCC.[53] It has been investigated in the adjuvant setting in a single-institution trial.[54] Patients with T2 (high-grade) to T4 or node-positive disease were randomized to thalidomide 300 mg daily for 2 years (n = 23) or observation (n = 23). The protocol was terminated early after a scheduled interim analysis showed that adjuvant thalidomide was unlikely to have the expected clinical benefit. Three-year recurrence-free survival was inferior in the thalidomide arm (28.7 vs 69.3%, $P = .022$). There was no difference in cancer-specific survival at 2 or 3 years.

Ongoing or Unreported Adjuvant Trials

Despite the host of negative adjuvant studies to date, there are numerous ongoing trials of adjuvant therapy using targeted agents, which are described in detail later. Five of the trials compare agents with proven activity in metastatic disease with placebo. ASSURE, S-TRAC, SORCE, and PROTECT compare adjuvant VEGF-targeted therapy with placebo, and EVEREST evaluates the role of adjuvant mammalian target of rapamycin (mTOR) inhibition. Although targeted agents might be effective in the adjuvant setting, some evidence suggests that they can adversely affect tumor biology, including promotion of tumor invasiveness and development of resistant metastases.[2,55–57] All of the trials are thus targeted at patients with high risk of recurrence, some using the predictive models described earlier. Both SORCE and EVEREST include patients with non-clear cell histology.[18]

ARISER

Girentuximab (Rencarex) is a chimeric monoclonal antibody against CA IX, also called the G250 antigen. CA IX is highly expressed on the cell surface of ccRCC. Girentuximab binds CA IX and is posited to induce antibody-dependent cellular cytotoxicity through natural killer cells and other immune effector cells. A double-blind, placebo-controlled phase III trial, Adjuvant Rencarex Immunotherapy Trial to Study Efficacy in Nonmetastatic RCC (ARISER), was undertaken to evaluate the impact of adjuvant girentuximab on the disease-free and overall survival of patients with ccRCC at high risk of recurrence (http://www.clinicaltrials.gov/; NCT00087022). A total of 864 patients with nonmetastatic high-grade T1b/T2, or T3-T4, or N+ ccRCC were randomized to weekly infusions of girentuximab or placebo for 24 weeks. Enrollment was completed in 2008. By January 2011, 340 recurrences had been reported.[18] In November 2011, in face of a declining recurrence rate, the Independent Data Monitoring Committee recommended terminating the interim analysis in favor of completing the final analysis, which is expected to be published in 2012.[58]

ASSURE

A phase III ECOG trial entitled Adjuvant Sorafenib or Sunitinib for Unfavorable Renal Carcinoma (ASSURE) has completed enrollment after enrolling more than 1900 patients (http://www.clinicaltrials.gov/; NCT00326898). Sorafenib (Nexavar) is an oral small molecule inhibitor of several tyrosine kinases, including Raf-kinase and VEGFR. Sunitinib (Sutent) is an oral small-molecule multityrosine kinase inhibitor of VEGFR, platelet-derived growth factor receptor (PDGFR), and KIT. Both sorafenib and sunitinib are active in mRCC.[59,60] Patients with nonmetastatic T1b (high-grade) to T4 or N+ RCC were randomized to up to 9 6-week courses of adjuvant sunitinib or sorafenib or placebo. The primary outcome is disease-free survival. Secondary end points include overall survival, safety, and molecular marker analyses. Although the study results are expected in April 2016, there has been concern regarding drug toxicity and early termination of therapy that may adversely influence trial outcome.

S-TRAC

Sunitinib is also being tested in an industry-sponsored phase III trial entitled Sunitinib Treatment of Renal Adjuvant Cancer (S-TRAC). Patients with high-risk ccRCC as defined by the UISS are being randomized to 1 year of sunitinib or placebo. Enrollment started in July 2007.

Estimated enrollment is 720 patients, with an anticipated completion in July 2017. The primary end point is disease-free survival. Secondary end points include overall survival, safety, and patient reported outcomes (http://www.clinicaltrials.gov/; NCT00375674).

SORCE

A Medical Research Council trial entitled A Phase III Randomised Double-Blind Study Comparing Sorafenib With Placebo in Patients With Resected Primary Renal Cell Carcinoma at High or Intermediate Risk of Relapse (SORCE) is ongoing in the United Kingdom (http://www.clinicaltrials.gov/; NCT00492258). Patients with RCC at intermediate or high risk of relapse (Leibovich score 3–11) are randomized after nephrectomy to placebo or 1 year of sorafenib or 3 years of sorafenib. The primary outcome is disease-free survival, with secondary outcomes including metastasis-free survival, overall survival, cost-effectiveness, and toxicity. Anticipated enrollment is 1656 patients. The final data for the primary result are expected to be collected in August 2012.

PROTECT

An industry-sponsored trial referred to as a Study to Evaluate Pazopanib as an Adjuvant Treatment for Localized RCC (PROTECT), is in progress (http://www.clinicaltrials.gov/; NCT01235962). Pazopanib (Votrient) is a potent multityrosine kinase inhibitor of VEGFR-1, VEGFR-2, VEGFR-3, PDGFR, and c-kit that is associated with improved progression-free survival in locally advanced and mRCC.[61] Patients with nonmetastatic T2 (high-grade) to T4 or N+ disease are being randomized after nephrectomy to 12 months of pazopanib or placebo. The primary outcome is disease-free survival. Overall survival is a secondary end point, along with safety and quality of life. Enrollment of the intended 1500 patients started in November 2010. The final data for the primary outcome will be collected in October 2015.

EVEREST

A Southwest Oncology Group (SWOG) trial called Everolimus for Renal Cancer Ensuing Surgical Therapy (EVEREST) is also currently enrolling participants (http://www.clinicaltrials.gov/; NCT01120249). Everolimus (Afinitor) is an mTOR inhibitor that has been shown to improve progression-free survival in patients with mRCC that has progressed on sunitinib or sorafenib.[62] Patients with nonmetastatic T1b (high-grade) to T4 or N+ RCC are randomized after nephrectomy to 9 courses of everolimus or placebo. The primary outcome is recurrence-free survival. Toxicity and overall survival are secondary end points.

Enrollment of an anticipated 1218 patients started in 2011. The final data for the primary result are expected to be collected in August 2013.

Adjuvant Therapy in Current Practice

There are no strong data to support the use of adjuvant therapy after nephrectomy for clinically localized disease. In randomized controlled trials, adjuvant radiotherapy, MPA, IL-2, IFN-α and thalidomide all showed no impact on disease progression or survival.[24,27,43–46,54,63] A single study, which has been criticized for methodological flaws, reported a large progression-free survival benefit with adjuvant autologous tumor vaccination.[48] Other vaccine studies failed in the adjuvant setting.[47,52] Ongoing studies of several tyrosine kinase inhibitors, an mTOR inhibitor, and a monoclonal antibody against CA IX are continuing the effort to decrease the risk of cancer recurrence and progression after nephrectomy for localized disease. The only accepted role for adjuvant therapy is in patients with high risk of recurrence in the setting of a research trial.

NEOADJUVANT THERAPY FOR LOCALLY ADVANCED RCC

Theoretic goals of neoadjuvant therapy for locally advanced RCC are to reduce the risk of recurrence, to shrink tumors to convert unresectable disease to resectable, to make partial nephrectomy feasible, or to simplify resection of a venous tumor thrombus. Although there is high-quality evidence in favor of neoadjuvant therapy in other genitourinary malignancies such as bladder, there are few data to guide the use of neoadjuvant systemic therapy in patients with nonmetastatic RCC.[64]

Immunotherapy

In metastatic disease, systemic immunotherapy is typically administered after cytoreductive nephrectomy because it has little or no impact on the primary lesion. In 16 patients with mRCC who were treated with neoadjuvant IL-2, IFN-α and granulocyte-macrophage colony-stimulating factor, no response was seen in the primary tumors.[65] Extrapolating to the neoadjuvant setting, cytokines are not expected to debulk nonmetastatic primary tumors effectively.[66]

On the other hand, neoadjuvant renal artery embolization (RAE) might provide some immunotherapeutic benefit because of release of tumor-associated antigens. In a case-control study, preoperative RAE was associated with improved overall survival at 5 years (62% vs 35%, $P = .01$)

and 10 years (47% vs 23%, *P* = .01), although this survival benefit has not been confirmed in a prospective trial.[67] It is possible that angioinfarction augments the immune response to the renal tumor.[68] There are reports of regression of RCC metastases after RAE and nephrectomy.[69,70] The postinfarction syndrome that is nearly universal may be cytokine mediated. Several studies have shown that RAE is immunomodulatory, with documented changes in natural killer cell activity, increased cell-mediated cytotoxicity, and alteration in lymphocyte proliferation.[71–73]

Targeted Therapy

Unlike immunotherapy, targeted therapies can have activity against the primary tumor.[74] This finding has prompted a reconsideration of the paradigm of neoadjuvant systemic therapy before surgical resection. This section focuses on neoadjuvant targeted therapy for nonmetastatic locally advanced disease, although some of the data are extrapolated from the presurgical (ie, metastatic) literature. The role of presurgical therapy before nephrectomy for metastatic disease is addressed later in the review.

Impact of targeted therapy on the primary tumor

Most of what is known about the impact of targeted therapy on the primary tumor is derived from studies of presurgical targeted therapy in the setting of metastatic disease. There are anecdotal reports of impressive responses in the primary tumor, including complete response, which is rare (**Fig. 3**).[75] Response in the primary tumor likely varies with each tumor and the systemic agent used.

Sunitinib has produced a higher rate of response than other targeted therapies.[18] In 2008, van der

Veldt and colleagues[76] reported a retrospective analysis of patients at 2 Dutch centers treated with sunitinib with the primary tumor in place from 2005 to 2007. Computed tomography (CT) scans were reviewed for effects on the primary tumor according to Response Evaluation Criteria in Solid Tumors (RECIST). Imaging was reviewed for 17 patients, 1 of whom had 2 primary lesions. According to RECIST, there were 4 partial responses, 1 progression, and 12 stable disease. In patients with partial response or stable disease by RECIST, the median reduction in tumor volume was 31% (*P* = .001), with an increase in the median volume of central necrosis of 39% (*P* = .035). RECIST criteria were not developed for use with targeted therapies such as angiogenesis inhibitors. The effect of targeted therapy may be associated with necrosis and cavitation rather than decrease in size, and is often underestimated by RECIST criteria.[77]

Similarly, in 2009, Thomas and colleagues[74] reported a retrospective series of 19 patients with locally advanced or mRCC who were treated with sunitinib with the primary tumor in place. Impact on the primary tumor was assessed by RECIST, with 3 partial responses (16%), 7 with stable disease (37%), and 9 (47%) with progression. Eight (42%) patients had tumor shrinkage, with a mean decrease of 24% (range 2%–46%).

Jonasch and colleagues[78] reported a prospective single-arm study of presurgical bevacizumab (n = 23) or bevacizumab plus erlotinib (n = 27) in patients with mRCC. Most patients (58%) had stable disease, with some partial responses (10%) and a single complete response (2%). Primary tumor regression was seen in 52% of patients and was modest: 1% to 10% shrinkage (29%), 11% to 20% shrinkage (16%), and 20% to 30% shrinkage (7%).

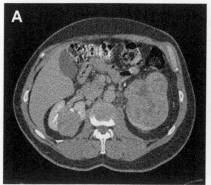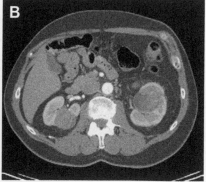

Fig. 3. A patient presented with extensive bilateral RCC, which was deemed unsuitable for resection (*A*). After 3 cycles of sunitinib, reduction in tumor burden permitted bilateral partial nephrectomy (*B*). (*Reprinted from Thomas AA, Rini BI, Stephenson AJ, et al. Surgical resection of renal cell carcinoma after targeted therapy. J Urol 2009;182:885; with permission.*)

Cowey and colleagues[79] performed a single-arm prospective study of neoadjuvant or presurgical sorafenib in patients with stage II or higher RCC in whom nephrectomy was planned. Thirty patients were treated for a median of 33 days. A total of 93% of patients had RECIST stable disease. There were no complete responses or progression by RECIST. Five patients had a measurable increase in the diameter of the primary, and the remainder had regression. The median change in tumor size was −9.6% (range +16 to −40%).

In 2011, Abel and colleagues[80] reported similarly modest changes in the primary tumor in a single-institution retrospective review of all patients with mRCC who received targeted therapy with the primary tumor in situ between November 2004 and December 2009. A total of 168 patients with adequate imaging were identified. Using RECIST criteria, 2 reviewers measured the diameter of primary and metastatic lesions on scans before and after targeted therapy. Median follow-up was 15 months. The median maximum initial primary tumor diameter was 9.6 cm. Patients received a variety of systemic targeted therapies (**Table 3**). The median maximum change in primary tumor diameter was −7.1% (interquartile range (IQR) −14.0 to −0.1) after a median 62 days (IQR 54–118) of treatment. The median change in primary tumor diameter was −6.5 mm (IQR −12.6 to −0.02).

Permitting resection

Although current targeted agents seem to have a modest impact on the size of the primary tumor, it has been proposed that neoadjuvant therapy may render initially unresectable lesions amenable to nephrectomy. Surgical resectability is a poorly defined, subjective characteristic.[66,81] Depending on the surgeon and patient, characteristics that may contribute to unresectability include tumor size, extensive hilar involvement, considerable lymphadenopathy, or adjacent organ invasion.[74] The series by Thomas and colleagues[74] included 4 patients without distant metastatic disease in whom the primary tumor was deemed unresectable because of proximity to adjacent structures (n = 4), bulky adenopathy (n = 2), and vascular involvement (n = 2). In these 4 patients, the average tumor size was 11.3 cm (range 6.4–20 cm). After neoadjuvant sunitinib, 3 of the 4 patients had tumor shrinkage (range 11%–24%) and were able to undergo resection. Other than tumor shrinkage, the changes that converted the tumors to resectable status were not characterized.

In the modern era, fewer than 1% of cases are deemed to be unresectable.[81] It is difficult to quantify the impact of neoadjuvant therapy on a phenomenon that is both rare and subjectively defined. With current drugs, in which striking responses in the primary are the exception rather than the rule, it is anticipated that conversion to resectability will remain a rare phenomenon.

Enabling nephron-sparing surgery

Most patients with renal cortical tumors have comorbid medicorenal disease.[82,83] Compared with partial nephrectomy, radical nephrectomy is associated with a higher risk of postoperative renal insufficiency.[84,85] There is a dose-response association between chronic kidney disease and

Table 3
In a retrospective review of all patients with mRCC who received targeted therapy with the primary tumor in situ, patients received a variety of systemic targeted therapies. Primary tumor response varied by drug

Agent	Number Patients (%)	Median Percentage Change (IQR)	Median Number Days Between Imaging (IQR)
Sunitinib	75 (45)	−10.2 (−21.1 to −2.8)	105 (76–201)
Bevacizumab	25 (15)	0.1 (−4.2 to 4.6)	55 (54–56)
Bevacizumab plus erlotinib	26 (15)	−10.1 (−17.1 to −6.0)	54.5 (54–56)
Sorafenib	16 (10)	−6.0 (−12.3 to 0.4)	90 (61.5–124)
Temsirolimus	16 (10)	−4.0 (−8.6 to −0.5)	56 (52–84)
Bevacizumab plus chemotherapy	7 (4)	−6.1 (−11.9 to −0.7)	58 (43–118)
Erlotinib	2 (1)	−5.1 (−9 to −1.3)	51.5 (41–62)
Pazopanib	1 (1)	−11.1 (NA)	48 (NA)

Data from Abel EJ, Culp SH, Tannir NM, et al. Primary tumor response to targeted agents in patients with metastatic renal cell carcinoma. Eur Urol 2011;59:10–5.

hospitalizations, cardiovascular events, and death.[86] In a study combining SEER (Surveillance Epidemiology and End Results) cancer registry data with Medicare claims, radical nephrectomy was associated with a 1.4-fold higher number of cardiovascular events (P<.05) and a higher risk of overall mortality (HR 1.38, P<.01) compared with partial nephrectomy.[87] Given the apparent benefits of nephron-sparing surgery, it has been proposed that neoadjuvant systemic therapy might enable partial nephrectomy when it would otherwise not be possible.[66,88]

The use of neoadjuvant targeted therapies to permit elective partial nephrectomy is not supported by evidence.[81] Neoadjuvant sunitinib has been used to enable imperative partial nephrectomy. A case was reported of a patient with 2 recurrences in the contralateral kidney after radical nephrectomy.[89] The lesions were not believed to be amenable to partial nephrectomy because of size and centrality. The tumors shrank 20% in association with neoadjuvant sunitinib, and subsequently were treated with partial nephrectomy. Similarly, Thomas and colleagues[90] reported 2 patients with extensive bilateral disease who were treated with neoadjuvant sunitinib to facilitate partial nephrectomy.

In 2010, Silberstein and colleagues[91] reported their experience with the use of neoadjuvant or presurgical sunitinib in 12 patients with 14 tumors before partial nephrectomy. In all patients, partial nephrectomy was deemed imperative because of renal insufficiency (n = 9), solitary kidney (n = 7), or bilateral tumors (n = 2). Five patients had metastatic disease. After sunitinib, the mean tumor diameter decreased from 7.1 cm to 5.6 cm (21%). All patients had measurable tumor shrinkage, but there were only 4 formal partial responses and no complete responses. All patients underwent nephron-sparing surgery. There were 3 urine leaks. Follow-up was 23.9 months. The study is hampered by several limitations, including absence of a control group, short follow-up, and lack of objective anatomic or morphometric data to quantify change in surgical complexity of the tumor (eg, centrality index or nephrometry score).[92,93] Most importantly, the indication for upfront sunitinib was not reported; the investigators do not state if partial nephrectomy would have been feasible without sunitinib.

Likewise, Hellenthal and colleagues[88] report a single-arm prospective study of neoadjuvant or presurgical sunitinib in 20 patients with localized or metastatic ccRCC. Seventeen of 20 patients (85%) had tumor shrinkage after 2 months of therapy, with a mean decrease of 11.8%. Twelve patients had radical nephrectomy. Eight had partial nephrectomy for pT1b to pT3a N0 M0 disease. No intraoperative or postoperative complications were attributed to the upfront targeted therapy. Although these series suggest that partial nephrectomy is feasible after sunitinib, they do not provide efficacy data to support the use of systemic therapy before partial nephrectomy.

Downsizing caval tumor thrombus

Neoadjuvant targeted therapy may have a role in downsizing caval tumor thrombus, but the supporting data are similarly problematic. In 2007, Karakiewicz and colleagues[94] reported a case of an 11-cm renal tumor with associated atrial thrombus. After the patient refused sternotomy, neoadjuvant sunitinib was successfully used to downsize the tumor thrombus. Twelve weeks after starting neoadjuvant therapy, the tumor thrombus was markedly smaller, protruding from the renal vein slightly into the infrahepatic inferior vena cava (Fig. 4). This situation permitted a less morbid surgical approach. Similarly, presurgical sunitinib has been used to shrink a caval thrombus to permit laparoscopic rather than open cytoreductive nephrectomy.[95]

Favorable responses in caval tumor thrombi are not universal. In 2010, Bex and colleagues[96] reported 2 patients with mRCC who received presurgical sunitinib in a phase II trial. One patient developed a new caval tumor thrombus and the second had extension of an existing infrahepatic thrombus up to the atrium despite presurgical sunitinib.

In the largest series to date, Cost and colleagues[97] reported on 25 patients with RCC who were treated with targeted therapy in the presence of a level 2 (n = 18), level 3 (n = 5), or level 4 (n = 2) venous tumor thrombus. Most of the patients (76%) had ccRCC. Initial systemic therapies were sunitinib (n = 12), bevacizumab (n = 9), temsirolimus (n = 3), and sorafenib (n = 1). A total of 36% of the patients were treated with radical nephrectomy and tumor thrombectomy after systemic therapy. In response to systemic therapy, thrombus height decreased in 44% of patients and increased in 28%. The thrombus level increased in 1 patient (level 2–3) and decreased in 3 patients (level 4 to 3, 3 to 2, and 2 to 0). The surgical approach would have been affected only in the patient with the regressed atrial thrombus. The limitations of the study include the retrospective design, heterogeneous patient population, variety of systemic therapies, and that not all patients were surgical candidates. Using systemic targeted therapy to

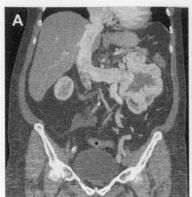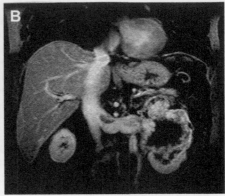

Fig. 4. (*A*) CT scan showing left-sided primary tumor with venous tumor thrombus extending into right atrium (*A*). After 2 cycles of sunitinib, the thrombus has regressed, visible as a dark filling defect at the junction of the left renal vein and inferior vena cava (*B*). (*Reprinted from* Karakiewicz PI, Suardi N, Jeldres C, et al. Neoadjuvant sutent induction therapy may effectively down-stage renal cell carcinoma atrial thrombi. Eur Urol 2008;53:846; with permission.)

shrink tumor thrombi before surgery needs further study and remains investigational.

Neoadjuvant Therapy in Current Practice

There is no strong direct evidence to support the use of neoadjuvant systemic therapy for locally advanced, nonmetastatic RCC. Systemic immunotherapy has little or no impact on the primary tumor, and is believed to work better after nephrectomy.[65] Although neoadjuvant RAE might initiate an antitumor immune response, the reported survival benefit has not been confirmed prospectively.[67] Although targeted therapies seem to be more apt to shrink the primary lesion than immunotherapy, the impact on the primary lesion seems to be modest and the potential benefits of neoadjuvant therapy (converting unresectable disease to resectable, facilitating nephron-sparing surgery, and shrinking venous tumor thrombus) remain theoretic. Clearly, further research is needed in this area to determine what, if any, benefit neoadjuvant approaches may have in the management of locally advanced RCC.

INTEGRATING SURGERY AND SYSTEMIC THERAPY IN METASTATIC DISEASE

RCC is unique among solid tumors, in that removal of the primary tumor is an essential component of the treatment of metastatic disease, even in asymptomatic patients.[5] The proper integration of cytoreductive surgery and systemic therapy remains to be elucidated with regards to selection of patients for cytoreduction, the role of cytoreduction in the era of targeted therapy, and the sequence of therapy.

Cytoreductive Nephrectomy

In the setting of metastatic disease, nephrectomy was formerly limited to palliation.[5] With the advent of systemic immunotherapy, cytoreductive nephrectomy was investigated as a therapeutic endeavor based on several observations. First, it was noted that the primary tumor had little or no response to systemic immunotherapy. In addition, it was noted that the primary tumor was associated with an inhibited immune response to the tumor and might act as a source for further metastatic progression.[98]

Several retrospective series of immunotherapy showed that previous nephrectomy was a favorable, independent prognostic factor.[99–103] In 1999, Motzer and colleagues[103] created a multivariate model to predict survival by analyzing 670 patients with advanced RCC who were treated from 1975 to 1996. In addition to Karnofsky performance status less than 80%, lactate dehydrogenase (LDH) level 1.5-fold greater than normal, low hemoglobin, and corrected serum calcium level greater than 10 mg/dL, absence of nephrectomy was an independent predictor of shorter survival.

Two randomized trials from SWOG and the European Organization for the Research and Treatment of Cancer (EORTC) were published in 2001 that evaluated the role of cytoreductive nephrectomy before systemic treatment with IFN-α in patients with mRCC.[104,105] The trials were similarly designed. Patients with a resectable tumor were randomized to cytoreductive nephrectomy followed by IFN-α versus IFN-α alone. Both trials reported improved overall survival, which was the primary end point, in the cytoreduction arm. In a combined analysis, cytoreductive nephrectomy followed by IFN-α was associated with longer median survival than IFN-α alone (13.6 vs 7.8 months, P = .002).[106] Based on these efforts, cytoreductive surgery before systemic therapy became the dominant treatment paradigm in mRCC.

Patient selection is paramount

Not all patients with mRCC benefit from cytoreductive nephrectomy. The risks of cytoreductive nephrectomy include cancer progression during recovery from surgery, surgical morbidity precluding patients from receiving systemic therapy, and delay in the initiation of systemic therapy to treat metastatic disease. When interpreting the SWOG and EORTC trials, it is essential to note their selection criteria. Patients were excluded from both trials for ECOG performance status of 2 or worse, previous systemic therapy, tumor thrombus above the renal veins, and unresectable primary before systemic therapy. In the EORTC trial, patients with brain metastases were also ineligible.

Several retrospective series identified clinical factors that were predictive of a favorable response to surgery.[5,98,107–111] Better outcomes were reported with good performance status, absence of central nervous system, liver or extensive bone metastases, absence of sarcomatoid or other poor prognosis histology, and debulking of a high fraction of disease.[5]

In 2010, Culp and colleagues[112] identified preoperative factors that were prognostic of cytoreductive nephrectomy outcome in mRCC. The investigators retrospectively compared patients who underwent cytoreductive nephrectomy (n = 566) with patients managed without cytoreduction (n = 110) from 1991 to 2007. Based on Kaplan-Meier analysis, the investigators determined that cytoreductive nephrectomy patients who died within 8.5 months of surgery did not receive a survival benefit from surgery compared with patients managed without surgery (P < .05). The surgical group was divided into 2 cohorts based on survival greater or less than 8.5 months. On multivariate analysis, independent predictors of inferior overall survival among cytoreductive nephrectomy patients were increased LDH level (HR 1.66, P <.001), low albumin level (HR 1.59, P = .001), symptomatic metastases at presentation (HR 1.35, P = .028), liver metastases (HR 1.47, P = .039), retroperitoneal adenopathy (HR 1.29, P = .040), supradiaphragmatic adenopathy (HR 1.48, P = .001), and clinical T3 (HR 1.37, P = .045) or T4 disease (HR 2.05, P = .019). Patients with 4 or more risk factors did not benefit

from cytoreductive nephrectomy; their survival curve was similar to that of patients treated with medical therapy alone (**Fig. 5**).

In the study by Culp and colleagues, fewer than 3% of patients had ECOG performance status 2; none had performance status 3 or greater. There were brain metastases in 3.5%. Thus, in a cohort of patients that seems largely similar to that of the ECOG and SWOG studies, this study shows a broad range of outcomes after cytoreductive nephrectomy. It emphasizes that not all candidates benefit from cytoreduction and identifies 7 clinical factors to select the patients most likely to benefit from extirpative surgery.

Targeted therapy: impact on the role of cytoreductive surgery

In accordance with the model established in the immunotherapy era, cytoreduction has remained an integral component of managing mRCC in the targeted therapy era. In the phase III trials reporting progression-free or overall survival advantages compared with control for sunitinib, sorafenib, temsirolimus, everolimus, bevacizumab/IFN-α2b, and bevacizumab/IFN-α2a, the rates of previous nephrectomy in the intervention arms were 91%, 94%, 66%, 96%, 85%, and 100%, respectively.[59,60,62,113–115] The lower rate of nephrectomy in the temsirolimus trial is explained by the proportion of high-risk patients in that trial.[113]

Despite the common use of cytoreductive nephrectomy, the benefit of integrating cytoreductive nephrectomy and targeted therapy nonetheless remains largely speculative. The means by

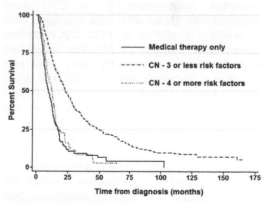

Fig. 5. Kaplan-Meier curve for overall survival after cytoreductive nephrectomy for mRCC based on number of preoperative risk factors. The curve for patients with 4 or more risk factors approximates that of patients treated with medical therapy alone. (*Reprinted from* Culp SH, Tannir NM, Abel EJ, et al. Can we better select patients with metastatic renal cell carcinoma for cytoreductive nephrectomy? Cancer 2010;116:3385; with permission.)

which cytoreduction improved survival in cytokine patients is unknown. In the combined analysis of the SWOG and EORTC immunotherapy trials, 253 patients had measurable disease.[106] In these 253 patients, objective response rates in the nephrectomy plus IFN and IFN alone groups were similarly low (6.9 vs 5.7%, P = .60). The mechanism by which cytoreduction improved survival in the absence of a measurable improvement in metastatic disease is unclear.[2,98] Mechanisms have been proposed including a tumoristatic effect of postnephrectomy azotemia and metabolic acidosis, improved immune surveillance after removal of the immunologic sink, and elimination of a source of growth factors.[2,98] It is possible that the observed benefit may not be inherent to the operation, but may be particular to the systemic agent used thereafter. The uncertain benefit of cytoreduction in the era of targeted therapy and the potential downsides of surgery, including disease progression during postoperative convalescence and surgical morbidity delaying or preventing administration of systemic therapy, have led to reevaluation of the paradigm of integrated therapy.

Several retrospective studies and subgroup analyses have confirmed the survival advantage of cytoreductive nephrectomy in the era of targeted therapy.[116–118] In a multicenter retrospective review, Choueri and colleagues[117] analyzed 645 patients treated with sunitinib, sorafenib, or bevacizumab between 2004 and 2008. Patients who underwent a primary (ie, noncytoreductive) nephrectomy with subsequent development of metastatic disease were excluded (n = 331). In the remaining population, patients who had cytoreductive nephrectomy (n = 201) were compared with those who were managed with the primary in situ (n = 113). Cytoreductive patients were younger (P<.01), less often had low performance status (P<.01), more often had more than 1 metastatic site (P = .04), less often received targeted therapy within a year of diagnosis (P<.01), and less often had hypercalcemia (P<.01). On multivariable analysis, cytoreductive nephrectomy was associated with improved overall survival (HR 0.68, P = .04). The survival benefit was marginal in patients with poor performance status and high-risk disease. Although the study is limited by possible selection bias inherent to retrospective analysis, it lends support to the continued use of cytoreduction in appropriate patients.[119]

An important phase III trial, the Clinical Trial to Assess the Importance of Nephrectomy (CARMENA), is ongoing in France and will help more rigorously establish whether or not cytoreductive nephrectomy before sunitinib is associated with improved survival (http://www.clinicaltrials.gov/; NCT00930033). Eligibility criteria include metastatic ccRCC, good performance status, and absence of brain metastases. A total of 576 patients will be randomized to cytoreductive nephrectomy followed by sunitinib or sunitinib alone. Enrollment started in 2009 and is anticipated to be completed in May 2013. The primary end point is overall survival. Secondary end points include objective response, progression-free survival, and postoperative morbidity.

The survival benefits of targeted therapeutics were reported primarily in patients who had previous cytoreductive nephrectomy. The highest quality data, albeit retrospective, suggest that cytoreductive nephrectomy in concert with targeted therapy is associated with improved survival compared with targeted therapy alone. For these reasons, cytoreductive nephrectomy is likely to remain a standard component of the treatment paradigm for appropriately selected patients pending the results of prospective studies such as CARMENA.[119–121]

Sequence of Therapy: the Role of Presurgical Targeted Therapy

Rationale for upfront targeted therapy

Unlike with immunotherapy, it is not clear that upfront surgery followed by targeted therapy will prove to be the best model.[5,120] Several advantages of presurgical targeted therapy have been proposed. Presurgical systemic therapy may reduce RCC-related morbidity before surgery.[120] In addition, nephrectomy specimens after presurgical treatment will be a valuable resource for molecular evaluation of mechanism of action and markers of response.[2,5]

Presurgical targeted therapy may also make the primary tumor more amenable to resection, as already discussed for locally advanced disease. van der Veldt and colleagues[76] reported 3 patients with metastatic disease and primaries that were believed to be unresectable because of suspected liver invasion. All went on to cytoreductive surgery after presurgical sunitinib and primary tumor volume reductions of 30% to 46%. In 2009, Bex and colleagues[122] published a retrospective analysis of 10 patients with mRCC who received sunitinib without previous nephrectomy because of doubtful resectability, defined as primary or retroperitoneal nodal masses invading adjacent organs or encasing vital structures such as the great vessels, celiac axis, or superior mesenteric artery. According to RECIST, there were 2 partial responses. The median change in the primary tumor was −10% (range −20 to +11%). The surgery-limiting tumor site diminished in 6 patients, most prominently in the first 2 to 4 months, which permitted cytoreductive nephrectomy in 3 patients. It seems that downsizing by current agents is limited in patients with mRCC and complex primary tumors.[2] Should presurgical therapy be adopted broadly, it will likely be because of other benefits unless future therapies are significantly more effective at downsizing the primary.

Perhaps most importantly, presurgical targeted therapy may act as a litmus test to select patients with stable or responsive disease for surgical consolidation.[5] It is theorized that those with rapidly progressive disease despite targeted therapy would be less likely to benefit from surgery and would instead go on to alternative systemic therapy.[5] There is indirect evidence to support this approach. In a multivariate analysis of long-term results from the SWOG trial, early disease progression within 90 days predicted overall survival (HR 2.1, $P<.0001$).[123] In the presurgical bevacizumab study by Jonasch and colleagues,[78] 6 patients (12%) had clinical or radiographic progression despite systemic therapy and, per protocol, did not go on to nephrectomy. All 6 patients were switched to alternative systemic therapies. None achieved disease stabilization or response. Sparing patients from needless surgery and its attendant risks is a beneficial goal of presurgical targeted therapy.

Evidence in favor of presurgical targeted therapy
Numerous case reports and retrospective series have been published reporting the feasibility of presurgical targeted therapy.[74,90,95,122,124–128] In addition, several prospective single-arm studies have reported the safety and efficacy of targeted agents before planned cytoreductive nephrectomy.[78,79,122,129]

In the phase II presurgical bevacizumab or bevacizumab plus erlotinib trial by Jonasch and colleagues, median progression-free survival was 11.0 months (95% CI, 5.5–15.6 months) and median overall survival was 25.4 months. These outcomes are comparable with postsurgical treatment. In 2011, Powles and colleagues[129] published their findings from 2 single-arm phase II trials of sunitinib (2 or 3 cycles) before cytoreductive nephrectomy in metastatic ccRCC. Seventeen patients (33%) had MSKCC poor-risk disease and the remainder had intermediate-risk disease. The median progression-free survival was 8 months (95% CI 5–15). Three patients (6%) had partial response by RECIST, and the median reduction in the primary tumor was 12% (range 8%–35%).

A total of 37 of 53 patients (70%) went on to cytoreductive nephrectomy. In some patients, surgery was not pursued because of disease progression (n = 9), patient preference (n = 3), and patient not fit for surgery (n = 2). No patients became ineligible for surgery because of local progression. Sunitinib was resumed postoperatively at a median of 21 days. Complications occurred in 27% of patients, including a postoperative death from respiratory failure.

Safety of presurgical targeted therapy
A strong evidence basis is essential because presurgical therapy is not without risk. Presurgical therapy is unproved compared with upfront cytoreductive nephrectomy, which has a survival benefit shown in randomized trials, albeit with different systemic agents. Arguments against presurgical therapy include possible adverse alterations in disease biology, including increased invasion, metastasis, and resistance.[2,55–57] In addition, presurgical therapy may affect wound healing and increase the complications associated with cytoreductive nephrectomy.[2] In a retrospective review, Chapin and colleagues evaluated all patients with mRCC who underwent cytoreductive nephrectomy at a single center from 2004 to 2010. Patients were treated with a variety of presurgical targeted agents including bevacizumab, bevacizumab plus erlotinib, sunitinib, sorafenib, erlotinib, and temsirolimus. Complications within 12 months of surgery were compared for patients who received presurgical systemic therapy (n = 70) and those who had immediate cytoreductive nephrectomy (n = 103). Complications were scored according to the Clavien-Dindo scale. Ninety-nine of 173 patients (57%) had 232 complications. Presurgical systemic targeted therapy was not associated with increased risk of overall or severe complications ($\geq$Clavien grade 3) on multivariable analysis. Patients treated with presurgical targeted therapy were more likely to have wound complications such as superficial wound dehiscence or infection (HR 4.14, $P = .003$).

Duration of presurgical targeted therapy
The proper duration of presurgical therapy is unclear and likely depends on a variety of factors, including drug and response to therapy. In 2011, Abel and colleagues[130] published a retrospective review of all mRCC patients at a single institution who were treated with sunitinib with the primary tumor in situ from 2004 to 2009. The median maximum overall change in the size of the primary tumor was −10.2%, which occurred at a median of 120 days after the start of systemic therapy. Early

tumor response, which was defined as a decrease of 10% or greater within 60 days, was an independent predictor of improved overall survival (HR 0.26, $P = .031$) on multivariate analysis. It seems that the effect of downsizing the primary tumor is most prominent in the first 2 to 4 months, which has been interpreted to mean that 3 cycles of presurgical sunitinib is sufficient.[2,76] Nonetheless, it is not yet clear that the proper duration of presurgical therapy will be dictated by the primary tumor response.

Ongoing or unreported presurgical trials

More than a dozen phase II trials are in progress investigating presurgical targeted therapy in advanced or mRCC, including evaluations of sorafenib, sunitinib, everolimus, pazopanib, and axitinib.[2,18] In addition, an important phase III EORTC trial is evaluating the proper sequence of cytoreduction and systemic targeted therapy, called Immediate Surgery or Surgery After Sunitinib Malate in Treating Patients with Metastatic Kidney Cancer (SURTIME) (http://www.clinicaltrials.gov/; NCT01099423). Patients with metastatic ccRCC with a resectable primary are being enrolled in Europe and Canada, and are randomized to immediate cytoreductive nephrectomy followed by sunitinib 4 weeks later, or 3 courses of presurgical sunitinib followed by cytoreductive nephrectomy. The primary end point is progression-free survival. Secondary end points include overall survival, morbidity, primary tumor response to sunitinib in the deferred surgery arm, and early progression. In a subset of patients, tissue will be collected at baseline and at surgery to evaluate differences in gene expression associated with sunitinib treatment. Enrollment of an estimated 458 patients commenced in April 2010. The final data for the primary end point are expected to be collected in October 2014. SURTIME is designed to address fundamental controversies in the treatment of mRCC, and along with CARMENA, SURTIME will advance our knowledge of the proper integration of systemic targeted therapy and cytoreductive nephrectomy.

Integration of CN and Systemic Therapy in Current Practice

The proper integration of cytoreductive surgery and systemic therapy is unclear. Correct selection of patients for cytoreduction, the role of cytoreduction in the era of targeted therapy, and the ideal sequence of therapy are ongoing topics of research. Clinical data should be used to select the patients most likely to benefit from extirpative surgery. Although a survival benefit has not been prospectively shown for cytoreductive

nephrectomy in the targeted therapy era, it is likely to remain a standard component of the treatment paradigm pending the results of prospective studies such as CARMENA and SURTIME.[119–121] Until the results of SURTIME are available, upfront cytoreductive nephrectomy in appropriately selected patients is likely to remain the default treatment algorithm, with presurgical targeted therapy an active focus of research.

SUMMARY

Proper integration of surgery and systemic therapy is essential for improving outcomes in RCC. Although there are no strong data to support the current use of adjuvant therapy after nephrectomy for clinically localized disease, ongoing studies of several tyrosine kinase inhibitors, an mTOR inhibitor, and a monoclonal antibody against CA IX are promising. Likewise, no strong direct evidence supports the use of neoadjuvant systemic therapy for locally advanced, nonmetastatic RCC. Although targeted therapies are more active against the primary tumor than immunotherapy, the impact on the primary lesion with current agents seems to be modest. The potential benefits of neoadjuvant therapy such as converting unresectable disease to resectable, facilitating nephron-sparing surgery, and shrinking venous tumor thrombus remain theoretic and are in need of further study. In metastatic disease, the proper integration of cytoreductive surgery and systemic therapy remains to be elucidated with regards to selection of patients for cytoreduction, the role of cytoreduction in the era of targeted therapy, and the ideal sequence of therapy. Presurgical targeted therapy is feasible and may be beneficial. Pending the results of randomized controlled trials, upfront cytoreductive nephrectomy in appropriate patients will continue as the paradigm of choice in mRCC.

REFERENCES

1. Howlader N, Noone A, Kraphcho M, et al, editors. SEER cancer statistics review, 1975-2008. 2011. Available at: http://seer.cancer.gov/csr/1975_2008/. Accessed December 7, 2011.
2. Bex A, Jonasch E, Kirkali Z, et al. Integrating surgery with targeted therapies for renal cell carcinoma: current evidence and ongoing trials. Eur Urol 2010;58:819–28.
3. Crispen PL, Boorjian SA, Lohse CM, et al. Predicting disease progression after nephrectomy for localized renal cell carcinoma: the utility of

prognostic models and molecular biomarkers. Cancer 2008;113:450–60.

4. Jacobsohn K, Wood C. Adjuvant therapy for renal cell carcinoma. Semin Oncol 2006;33:576–82.

5. Wood CG. Multimodal approaches in the management of locally advanced and metastatic renal cell carcinoma: combining surgery and systemic therapies to improve patient outcome. Clin Cancer Res 2007;13:697s–702s.

6. Kattan MW, Reuter V, Motzer RJ, et al. A postoperative prognostic nomogram for renal cell carcinoma. J Urol 2001;166:63–7.

7. Sorbellini M, Kattan MW, Snyder ME, et al. A postoperative prognostic nomogram predicting recurrence for patients with conventional clear cell renal cell carcinoma. J Urol 2005;173:48–51.

8. Leibovich BC, Blute ML, Cheville JC, et al. Prediction of progression after radical nephrectomy for patients with clear cell renal cell carcinoma: a stratification tool for prospective clinical trials. Cancer 2003;97:1663–71.

9. Zisman A. Risk group assessment and clinical outcome algorithm to predict the natural history of patients with surgically resected renal cell carcinoma. J Clin Oncol 2002;20:4559–66.

10. Levy DA, Slaton JW, Swanson DA, et al. Stage specific guidelines for surveillance after radical nephrectomy for local renal cell carcinoma. J Urol 1998;159:1163–7.

11. Klatte T, Lam JS, Shuch B, et al. Surveillance for renal cell carcinoma: why and how? When and how often? Urol Oncol 2008;26:550–4.

12. Patard JJ. Use of the University of California Los Angeles integrated staging system to predict survival in renal cell carcinoma: an international multicenter study. J Clin Oncol 2004;22:3316–22.

13. Lane BR, Kattan MW. Prognostic models and algorithms in renal cell carcinoma. Urol Clin North Am 2008;35:613–25, vii.

14. Cindolo L, Patard J-J, Chiodini P, et al. Comparison of predictive accuracy of four prognostic models for nonmetastatic renal cell carcinoma after nephrectomy: a multicenter European study. Cancer 2005;104:1362–71.

15. Cindolo L, la Taille de A, Messina G, et al. A preoperative clinical prognostic model for nonmetastatic renal cell carcinoma. BJU Int 2003;92:901–5.

16. Yaycioglu O, Roberts WW, Chan T, et al. Prognostic assessment of nonmetastatic renal cell carcinoma: a clinically based model. Urology 2001;58:141–5.

17. Raj GV, Thompson RH, Leibovich BC, et al. Preoperative nomogram predicting 12-year probability of metastatic renal cancer. J Urol 2008;179:2146–51 [discussion: 2151].

18. Smaldone MC, Fung C, Uzzo RG, et al. Adjuvant and neoadjuvant therapies in high-risk renal cell carcinoma. Hematol Oncol Clin North Am 2011; 25:765–91.

19. Kim HL. Using protein expressions to predict survival in clear cell renal carcinoma. Clin Cancer Res 2004;10:5464–71.

20. Klatte T, Seligson DB, LaRochelle J, et al. Molecular signatures of localized clear cell renal cell carcinoma to predict disease-free survival after nephrectomy. Cancer Epidemiol Biomarkers Prev 2009;18:894–900.

21. Parker AS, Leibovich BC, Lohse CM, et al. Development and evaluation of BioScore: a biomarker panel to enhance prognostic algorithms for clear cell renal cell carcinoma. Cancer 2009;115:2092–103.

22. Choueiri M, Tannir N, Jonasch E. Adjuvant and neoadjuvant therapy in renal cell carcinoma. Curr Clin Pharmacol 2011;6:144–50.

23. Aref I, Bociek RG, Salhani D. Is post-operative radiation for renal cell carcinoma justified? Radiother Oncol 1997;43:155–7.

24. Finney R. The value of radiotherapy in the treatment of hypernephroma–a clinical trial. BJU Int 1973;45: 258–69.

25. Kjaer M, Frederiksen P. Postoperative radiotherapy in stage II and III renal adenocarcinoma. A randomized trial by the Copenhagen renal cancer study group. Int J Radiat Oncol Biol Phys 1987; 13:665–72.

26. Lam JS, Belldegrun AS, Figlin RA. Adjuvant treatment for renal cell carcinoma. Expert Opin Pharmacother 2006;7:706–20.

27. Pizzocaro G, Piva L, Di Fronzo G, et al. Adjuvant medroxyprogesterone acetate to radical nephrectomy in renal cancer: 5-year results of a prospective randomized study. J Urol 1987;138:1379–81.

28. Shimabukuro T, Naito K. Tumor-infiltrating lymphocytes derived from human renal cell carcinoma: clonal analysis of its characteristics. Int J Urol 2008;15:241–4.

29. Kradin R, Lazarus D, Dubinett S, et al. Tumour-infiltrating lymphocytes and interleukin-2 in treatment of advanced cancer. Lancet 1989;333:577–80.

30. Finke J, Tubbs R, Connelly B, et al. Tumor-infiltrating lymphocytes in patients with renal-cell carcinoma. Ann N Y Acad Sci 1988;532:387–94.

31. Vogelzang NJ, Priest ER, Borden L. Spontaneous regression of histologically proved pulmonary metastases from renal cell carcinoma: a case with 5-year followup. J Urol 1992;148:1247–8.

32. Sánchez-Ortiz RF, Tannir N, Ahrar K, et al. Spontaneous regression of pulmonary metastases from renal cell carcinoma after radio frequency ablation of primary tumor: an in situ tumor vaccine? J Urol 2003;170:178–9.

33. Fujikawa K, Matsui Y, Miura K, et al. Serum immunosuppressive acidic protein and natural killer

cell activity in patients with metastatic renal cell carcinoma before and after nephrectomy. J Urol 2000;164:673–5.

34. Dadian G, Riches PG, Henderson DC, et al. Immunological parameters in peripheral blood of patients with renal cell carcinoma before and after nephrectomy. Br J Urol 1994;74:15–22.

35. Montie JE, Straffon RA, Deodhar SD, et al. In vitro assessment of cell-mediated immunity in patients with renal cell carcinoma. J Urol 1976;115:239–42.

36. Rayman P. Effect of renal cell carcinomas on the development of type 1 T-cell responses. Clin Cancer Res 2004;10:6360S–6S.

37. Arya M, Chao D, Patel HR. Allogeneic hematopoietic stem-cell transplantation: the next generation of therapy for metastatic renal cell cancer. Nat Clin Pract Oncol 2004;1:32–8.

38. McDermott DF, Regan MM, Clark JI, et al. Randomized phase III trial of high-dose interleukin-2 versus subcutaneous interleukin-2 and interferon in patients with metastatic renal cell carcinoma. J Clin Oncol 2005;23:133–41.

39. Lam J, Leppert J, Belldegrun A. Novel approaches in the therapy of metastatic renal cell carcinoma. World J Urol 2005;23:202–12.

40. Interferon-alpha and survival in metastatic renal carcinoma: early results of a randomised controlled trial. Medical Research Council Renal Cancer Collaborators. Lancet 1999;353:14–7.

41. Pyrhönen S, Salminen E, Ruutu M, et al. Prospective randomized trial of interferon alfa-2a plus vinblastine versus vinblastine alone in patients with advanced renal cell cancer. J Clin Oncol 1999;17:2859–67.

42. Fyfe G, Fisher RI, Rosenberg SA, et al. Results of treatment of 255 patients with metastatic renal cell carcinoma who received high-dose recombinant interleukin-2 therapy. J Clin Oncol 1995;13:688–96.

43. Messing EM, Manola J, Wilding G, et al. Phase III study of interferon alfa-NL as adjuvant treatment for resectable renal cell carcinoma: an Eastern Cooperative Oncology Group/Intergroup trial. J Clin Oncol 2003;21:1214–22.

44. Pizzocaro G, Piva L, Colavita M, et al. Interferon adjuvant to radical nephrectomy in Robson stages II and III renal cell carcinoma: a multicentric randomized study. J Clin Oncol 2001;19:425–31.

45. Clark JI, Atkins MB, Urba WJ, et al. Adjuvant high-dose bolus interleukin-2 for patients with high-risk renal cell carcinoma: a cytokine working group randomized trial. J Clin Oncol 2003;21:3133–40.

46. Atzpodien J, Schmitt E, Gertenbach U, et al. Adjuvant treatment with interleukin-2- and interferon-alpha2a-based chemoimmunotherapy in renal cell carcinoma post tumour nephrectomy: results of a prospectively randomised trial of the German

Cooperative Renal Carcinoma Chemoimmunotherapy Group (DGCIN). Br J Cancer 2005;92:843–6.

47. Galligioni E, Quaia M, Merlo A, et al. Adjuvant immunotherapy treatment of renal carcinoma patients with autologous tumor cells and bacillus Calmette-Guèrin: five-year results of a prospective randomized study. Cancer 1996;77:2560–6.

48. Jocham D, Richter A, Hoffmann L, et al. Adjuvant autologous renal tumour cell vaccine and risk of tumour progression in patients with renal-cell carcinoma after radical nephrectomy: phase III, randomised controlled trial. Lancet 2004;363:594–9.

49. Rassweiler J. Re: ten-year survival analysis for renal carcinoma patients treated with an autologous tumour lysate vaccine in an adjuvant setting. Eur Urol 2012;61:219–20.

50. Doehn C, Richter A, Theodor RA, et al. An adjuvant vaccination with Reniale prolongs survival in patients with renal cell carcinoma following radical nephrectomy. Eur Urol Suppl 2006;5:286. Available at: http://www.sciencedirect.com/science/article/pii/S0302283811011201. Accessed December 7, 2011.

51. May M, Brookman-May S, Hoschke B, et al. Ten-year survival analysis for renal carcinoma patients treated with an autologous tumour lysate vaccine in an adjuvant setting. Cancer Immunol Immunother 2010;59:687–95.

52. Wood C, Srivastava P, Bukowski R, et al. An adjuvant autologous therapeutic vaccine (HSPPC-96; vitespen) versus observation alone for patients at high risk of recurrence after nephrectomy for renal cell carcinoma: a multicentre, open-label, randomised phase III trial. Lancet 2008;372:145–54.

53. Daliani DD, Papandreou CN, Thall PF, et al. A pilot study of thalidomide in patients with progressive metastatic renal cell carcinoma. Cancer 2002;95:758–65.

54. Margulis V, Matin SF, Tannir N, et al. Randomized trial of adjuvant thalidomide versus observation in patients with completely resected high-risk renal cell carcinoma. Urology 2009;73:337–41.

55. Plimack ER, Tannir N, Lin E, et al. Patterns of disease progression in metastatic renal cell carcinoma patients treated with antivascular agents and interferon: impact of therapy on recurrence patterns and outcome measures. Cancer 2009;115:1859–66.

56. Ebos JML, Lee CR, Cruz-Munoz W, et al. Accelerated metastasis after short-term treatment with a potent inhibitor of tumor angiogenesis. Cancer Cell 2009;15:232–9.

57. Pàez-Ribes M, Allen E, Hudock J, et al. Antiangiogenic therapy elicits malignant progression of tumors to increased local invasion and distant metastasis. Cancer Cell 2009;15:220–31.

58. Arnold K. WILEX AG press release: ARISER Independent Data Monitoring Committee (IDMC)

recommends conducting the final analysis of the pivotal Phase III trial with RENCAREX. 2011. Available at: http://www.wilex.de/press-investors/announcements/press-releases/21112011-2/. Accessed December 7, 2011.

59. Escudier B, Eisen T, Stadler W. Sorafenib in advanced clear-cell renal-cell carcinoma. N Engl J Med 2007;356:125–34.

60. Motzer RJ, Hutson TE, Tomczak P, et al. Sunitinib versus interferon alfa in metastatic renal-cell carcinoma. N Engl J Med 2007;356:115–24.

61. Sternberg CN, Davis ID, Mardiak J, et al. Pazopanib in locally advanced or metastatic renal cell carcinoma: results of a randomized phase III trial. J Clin Oncol 2010;28:1061–8.

62. Motzer RJ, Escudier B, Oudard S, et al. Efficacy of everolimus in advanced renal cell carcinoma: a double-blind, randomised, placebo-controlled phase III trial. Lancet 2008;372:449–56.

63. Kjaer M, Iversen P, Hvidt V, et al. A randomized trial of postoperative radiotherapy versus observation in stage II and III renal adenocarcinoma. A study by the Copenhagen Renal Cancer Study Group. Scand J Urol Nephrol 1987;21(4):285–9.

64. Advanced Bladder Cancer Overview Collaboration. Neoadjuvant chemotherapy for invasive bladder cancer. Cochrane Database Syst Rev 2005;2:CD005246.

65. Bex A, Horenblas S, Meinhardt W, et al. The role of initial immunotherapy as selection for nephrectomy in patients with metastatic renal cell carcinoma and the primary tumor in situ. Eur Urol 2002;42:570–4 [discussion: 575–6].

66. Jonasch E, Tannir NM. Targeted therapy for locally advanced renal cell carcinoma. Target Oncol 2010; 5:113–8.

67. Zielinski H, Szmigielski S, Petrovich Z. Comparison of preoperative embolization followed by radical nephrectomy with radical nephrectomy alone for renal cell carcinoma. Am J Clin Oncol 2000;23:6–12.

68. Kalman D, Varenhorst E. The role of arterial embolization in renal cell carcinoma. Scand J Urol Nephrol 1999;33:162–70.

69. Mohr SJ, Whitesel JA. Spontaneous regression of renal cell carcinoma metastases after preoperative embolization of primary tumor and subsequent nephrectomy. Urology 1979;14:5–8.

70. Swanson DA, Johnson DE, Eschenbach von AC, et al. Angioinfarction plus nephrectomy for metastatic renal cell carcinoma–an update. J Urol 1983;130:449–52.

71. Bakke A, Göthlin JH, Haukaas SA, et al. Augmentation of natural killer cell activity after arterial embolization of renal carcinomas. Cancer Res 1982;42:3880–3.

72. Nakano H, Nihira H, Toge T. Treatment of renal cancer patients by transcatheter embolization and its effects on lymphocyte proliferative responses. J Urol 1983;130:24–7.

73. Johnson G, Kalland T. Enhancement of mouse natural killer cell activity after dearterialization of experimental renal tumors. J Urol 1984;132:1250–3.

74. Thomas AA, Rini BI, Lane BR, et al. Response of the primary tumor to neoadjuvant sunitinib in patients with advanced renal cell carcinoma. J Urol 2009;181:518–23 [discussion: 523].

75. Robert G, Gabbay G, Bram R, et al. Complete histologic remission after sunitinib neoadjuvant therapy in T3b renal cell carcinoma. Eur Urol 2009;55:1477–80.

76. Van der Veldt AA, Meijerink MR, van den Eertwegh AJ, et al. Sunitinib for treatment of advanced renal cell cancer: primary tumor response. Clin Cancer Res 2008;14:2431–6.

77. Desar IM, van Herpen CM, van Laarhoven HW, et al. Beyond RECIST: molecular and functional imaging techniques for evaluation of response to targeted therapy. Cancer Treat Rev 2009;35:309–21.

78. Jonasch E, Wood CG, Matin SF, et al. Phase II presurgical feasibility study of bevacizumab in untreated patients with metastatic renal cell carcinoma. J Clin Oncol 2009;27:4076–81.

79. Cowey CL, Amin C, Pruthi RS, et al. Neoadjuvant clinical trial with sorafenib for patients with stage II or higher renal cell carcinoma. J Clin Oncol 2010;28:1502–7.

80. Abel EJ, Culp SH, Tannir NM, et al. Primary tumor response to targeted agents in patients with metastatic renal cell carcinoma. Eur Urol 2011;59:10–5.

81. Ficarra V, Novara G. Kidney cancer: neoadjuvant targeted therapies in renal cell carcinoma. Nat Rev Urol 2010;7:63–4.

82. Bijol V, Mendez GP, Hurwitz S, et al. Evaluation of the nonneoplastic pathology in tumor nephrectomy specimens: predicting the risk of progressive renal failure. Am J Surg Pathol 2006;30:575–84.

83. Huang WC, Levey AS, Serio AM, et al. Chronic kidney disease after nephrectomy in patients with renal cortical tumours: a retrospective cohort study. Lancet Oncol 2006;7:735–40.

84. Lau WK, Blute ML, Weaver AL, et al. Matched comparison of radical nephrectomy vs nephron-sparing surgery in patients with unilateral renal cell carcinoma and a normal contralateral kidney. Mayo Clin Proc 2000;75:1236–42.

85. McKiernan J, Simmons R, Katz J, et al. Natural history of chronic renal insufficiency after partial and radical nephrectomy. Urology 2002;59:816–20.

86. Go AS, Chertow GM, Fan D, et al. Chronic kidney disease and the risks of death, cardiovascular events, and hospitalization. N Engl J Med 2004; 351:1296–305.

87. Huang WC, Elkin EB, Levey AS, et al. Partial nephrectomy versus radical nephrectomy in patients with small renal tumors–is there a difference in mortality and cardiovascular outcomes? J Urol 2009;181:55–61 [discussion: 61–2].

88. Hellenthal NJ, Underwood W, Penetrante R, et al. Prospective clinical trial of preoperative sunitinib in patients with renal cell carcinoma. J Urol 2010; 184:859–64.

89. Ansari J, Doherty A, McCafferty I, et al. Neoadjuvant sunitinib facilitates nephron-sparing surgery and avoids long-term dialysis in a patient with metachronous contralateral renal cell carcinoma. Clin Genitourin Cancer 2009;7:E39–41.

90. Thomas AA, Rini BI, Stephenson AJ, et al. Surgical resection of renal cell carcinoma after targeted therapy. J Urol 2009;182:881–6.

91. Silberstein JL, Millard F, Mehrazin R, et al. Feasibility and efficacy of neoadjuvant sunitinib before nephron-sparing surgery. BJU Int 2010; 106:1270–6.

92. Simmons MN, Ching CB, Samplaski MK, et al. Kidney tumor location measurement using the C index method. J Urol 2010;183:1708–13.

93. Kutikov A, Uzzo RG. The R.E.N.A.L. nephrometry score: a comprehensive standardized system for quantitating renal tumor size, location and depth. J Urol 2009;182:844–53.

94. Karakiewicz PI, Suardi N, Jeldres C, et al. Neoadjuvant sutent induction therapy may effectively downstage renal cell carcinoma atrial thrombi. Eur Urol 2008;53:845–8.

95. Harshman LC, Srinivas S, Kamaya A, et al. Laparoscopic radical nephrectomy after shrinkage of a caval tumor thrombus with sunitinib. Nat Rev Urol 2009;6:338–43.

96. Bex A, Van der Veldt AA, Blank C, et al. Progression of a caval vein thrombus in two patients with primary renal cell carcinoma on pretreatment with sunitinib. Acta Oncol 2010;49:520–3.

97. Cost N, Delacroix S Jr, Sleeper J, et al. The impact of targeted molecular therapies on the level of renal cell carcinoma vena caval tumor thrombus. Eur Urol 2011;59(6):912–8.

98. Flanigan RC. Debulking nephrectomy in metastatic renal cancer. Clin Cancer Res 2004;10:6335S–41S.

99. Mani S, Todd MB, Katz K, et al. Prognostic factors for survival in patients with metastatic renal cancer treated with biological response modifiers. J Urol 1995;154:35–40.

100. Fisher R, Coltman C. Metastatic renal cancer treated with interleukin-2 and lymphokine-activated killer cells. Ann Intern Med 1988;108:518–23.

101. Muss H, Costanzi J, Leavitt R. Recombinant alfa interferon in renal cell carcinoma: a randomized trial of two routes of administration. J Clin Oncol 1987;5:286–91.

102. Motzer RJ, Russo P. Systemic therapy for renal cell carcinoma. J Urol 2000;163:408–17.

103. Motzer RJ, Mazumdar M, Bacik J, et al. Survival and prognostic stratification of 670 patients with advanced renal cell carcinoma. J Clin Oncol 1999;17:2530–40.

104. Flanigan R, Salmon S. Nephrectomy followed by interferon alfa-2b compared with interferon alfa-2b alone for metastatic renal-cell cancer. N Engl J Med 2001;345:1655–9.

105. Mickisch GH, Garin A, van Poppel H, et al. Radical nephrectomy plus interferon-alfa-based immunotherapy compared with interferon alfa alone in metastatic renal-cell carcinoma: a randomised trial. Lancet 2001;358:966–70.

106. Flanigan RC, Mickisch G, Sylvester R, et al. Cytoreductive nephrectomy in patients with metastatic renal cancer: a combined analysis. J Urol 2004; 171:1071–6.

107. Pantuck AJ, Zisman A, Dorey F, et al. Renal cell carcinoma with retroperitoneal lymph nodes. Impact on survival and benefits of immunotherapy. Cancer 2003;97:2995–3002.

108. Vasselli JR, Yang JC, Linehan WM, et al. Lack of retroperitoneal lymphadenopathy predicts survival of patients with metastatic renal cell carcinoma. J Urol 2001;166:68–72.

109. Han K, Pantuck A, Bui M, et al. Number of metastatic sites rather than location dictates overall survival of patients with node-negative metastatic renal cell carcinoma. Urology 2003; 61(2):314–9.

110. Slaton J, Perrotte P, Balbay M, et al. Reassessment of the selection criteria for cytoreductive nephrectomy in patients with metastatic renal cell carcinoma. J Urol 2000;163:70.

111. Wood C, Huber N, Madsen L, et al. Clinical variables that predict survival following cytoreductive nephrectomy for metastatic renal cell carcinoma. J Urol 2001;165:184A.

112. Culp SH, Tannir NM, Abel EJ, et al. Can we better select patients with metastatic renal cell carcinoma for cytoreductive nephrectomy? Cancer 2010;116: 3378–88.

113. Hudes G, Carducci M, Tomczak P, et al. Temsirolimus, interferon alfa, or both for advanced renal-cell carcinoma. N Engl J Med 2007;356:2271–81.

114. Rini BI, Halabi S, Rosenberg JE, et al. Bevacizumab plus interferon alfa compared with interferon alfa monotherapy in patients with metastatic renal cell carcinoma: CALGB 90206. J Clin Oncol 2008; 26:5422–8.

115. Escudier B, Pluzanska A, Koralewski P, et al. Bevacizumab plus interferon alfa-2a for treatment of metastatic renal cell carcinoma: a randomised, double-blind phase III trial. Lancet 2007;370: 2103–11.

116. Szczylik C, Porta C, Bracarda S, et al. Sunitinib in patients with or without prior nephrectomy (Nx) in an expanded access trial of metastatic renal cell carcinoma (mRCC). J Clin Oncol 2008; 26 [abstr 5124]. Available at: http://meeting.asco-pubs.org/cgi/content/abstract/26/15_suppl/5124?sid=ee6c06b3-e9fb-4158-a5e5-54d5bddbfe40. Accessed December 9, 2011.

117. Choueiri TK, Xie W, Kollmannsberger C, et al. The impact of cytoreductive nephrectomy on survival of patients with metastatic renal cell carcinoma receiving vascular endothelial growth factor targeted therapy. J Urol 2011;185:60–6.

118. Warren M, Venner PM, North S, et al. A population-based study examining the effect of tyrosine kinase inhibitors on survival in metastatic renal cell carcinoma in Alberta and the role of nephrectomy prior to treatment. Can Urol Assoc J 2009;3:281–9.

119. Singer EA, Srinivasan R, Bratslavsky G. Editorial comment. J Urol 2011;185:66.

120. Margulis V, Wood CG. Cytoreductive nephrectomy in the era of targeted molecular agents: is it time to consider presurgical systemic therapy? Eur Urol 2008;54:489–92.

121. Margulis V, Wood CG, Jonasch E, et al. Current status of debulking nephrectomy in the era of tyrosine kinase inhibitors. Curr Oncol Rep 2008;10:253–8.

122. Bex A, Van der Veldt AA, Blank C, et al. Neoadjuvant sunitinib for surgically complex advanced renal cell cancer of doubtful resectability: initial experience with downsizing to reconsider cytoreductive surgery. World J Urol 2009;27:533–9.

123. Lara PN, Tangen CM, Conlon SJ, et al. Predictors of survival of advanced renal cell carcinoma: long-term results from Southwest Oncology Group Trial S8949. J Urol 2009;181:512–6 [discussion: 516–7].

124. Rodríguez Faba O, Breda A, Rosales A, et al. Neoadjuvant temsirolimus effectiveness in downstaging advanced non-clear cell renal cell carcinoma. Eur Urol 2010;58:307–10.

125. Shuch B, Riggs SB, LaRochelle JC, et al. Neoadjuvant targeted therapy and advanced kidney cancer: observations and implications for a new treatment paradigm. BJU Int 2008;102:692–6.

126. Amin C, Wallen E, Pruthi RS, et al. Preoperative tyrosine kinase inhibition as an adjunct to debulking nephrectomy. Urology 2008;72:864–8.

127. Wood CG, Margulis V. Neoadjuvant (presurgical) therapy for renal cell carcinoma: a new treatment paradigm for locally advanced and metastatic disease. Cancer 2009;115:2355–60.

128. Patard J-J, Thuret R, Raffi A, et al. Treatment with sunitinib enabled complete resection of massive lymphadenopathy not previously amenable to excision in a patient with renal cell carcinoma. Eur Urol 2009;55:237–9 [quiz: 239].

129. Powles T, Kayani I, Blank C, et al. The safety and efficacy of sunitinib before planned nephrectomy in metastatic clear cell renal cancer. Ann Oncol 2011;22:1041–7.

130. Abel EJ, Culp SH, Tannir NM, et al. Early primary tumor size reduction is an independent predictor of improved overall survival in metastatic renal cell carcinoma patients treated with sunitinib. Eur Urol 2011;60(6):1273–9.

Defining an Individualized Treatment Strategy for Metastatic Renal Cancer

Brian Hu, MD[a],*, Primo N. Lara Jr, MD[b],
Christopher P. Evans, MD[a]

KEYWORDS

- Renal cell carcinoma • Metastatic • Targeted therapy
- Individual • Personalize

One of 3 cases of renal cell carcinoma (RCC) is diagnosed with metastases at the time of initial presentation. In addition, 20% to 40% of patients treated for local disease experience metachronous metastases.[1] Once RCC has metastasized, the chance of durable complete response is low. Because RCC is traditionally viewed as chemotherapy resistant and radiotherapy resistant, early treatments relied on cytokine therapy, which had low response rates and high levels of treatment-related toxicity. Over the past 6 years, the armamentarium for treating metastatic RCC (mRCC) has increased greatly with the emergence of targeted therapy directed against angiogenesis and mammalian target of rapamycin (mTOR) pathways.

There are several factors that make treatment of mRCC well suited for an individualized approach. The first is its biologic diversity. The variability in response rates exemplifies differences in both tumor biology and host response to the tumor and therapy. Second, improvements are being made in the ability to recognize individual differences in mRCC, both clinical and molecular. Lastly, therapies against mRCC are numerous, allowing for adjustment of treatment.

The personalized approach to cancer therapy is based on the specific biology of either the tumor or the host. An example of this type of care is the use of HER2/neu in breast cancer. Patients who have expression of this receptor are treated with a monoclonal antibody against HER2/neu, which has been shown to improve survival. This approach to treating cancer offers more efficacious therapy while limiting the treatment-related toxicity in nonresponders.

This article addresses the improved understanding of RCC biology and the molecular pathways involved in tumorigenesis, reviews available surgical and systemic therapies as well as risk stratification tools and biomarkers that assist in prognostication and prediction of response, and, lastly, reviews the available data that can guide systemic therapy and surgery to a more individualized strategy.

RELEVANT BIOLOGIC PATHWAYS IN RCC

Tumor hypoxia is a common feature in solid tumors, such as RCC, and is associated with poor patient outcomes. Hypoxia is important in tumor progression because it has the potential to limit cell proliferation and differentiation while promoting necrosis and apoptosis.[2] Its presence can also lead to more aggressive tumors with

[a] Department of Urology, University of California, Davis, Medical Center, 4860 Y Street, Suite 3500, Sacramento, CA 95817, USA
[b] Division of Hematology and Oncology, Department of Internal Medicine, School of Medicine, University of California, Davis, 4501 X Street, Sacramento, CA 95817, USA
* Corresponding author.
E-mail address: Brian.hu@ucdmc.ucdavis.edu

Urol Clin N Am 39 (2012) 233–249
doi:10.1016/j.ucl.2012.02.002
0094-0143/12/$ – see front matter © 2012 Elsevier Inc. All rights reserved.

urologic.theclinics.com

abundant angiogenesis. RCC is a tumor that is known for its marked vascularity, and investigation into its biology has uncovered hypoxia-induced signaling as a main element in tumorigenesis and progression. **Fig. 1** provides an overview of the biologic pathways in RCC.[3]

Important in understanding the angiogenesis pathway for RCC is the identification of the von Hippel-Lindau (*VHL*) gene as a critical modulator of hypoxia-responsive gene elements. *VHL* is a tumor suppressor gene that encodes for the VHL protein. This protein complexes with cullin 2, elongin B, and elongin C to form the E3 ubiquitin-ligase complex.[4–6] In normoxic conditions, the ubiquitin-ligase complex targets hypoxia-inducible factors (HIF-1α and HIF-2α) for ubiquitin-mediated degradation by hydroxylation.[7] In hypoxic conditions, HIF-1α and HIF-2α do not undergo hydroxylation and act as transcription factors for more than 200 genes. Proteins regulated by HIF include vascular endothelial growth factor (VEGF) and platelet-derived growth factor (PDGF). Mutation of the both *VHL* genes causes defective complex formation. With an ineffective ubiquitin-ligase complex, HIF levels accumulate and facilitate the transcription of genes involved in angiogenesis, cell survival, and cell proliferation.[8]

HIF can receive input from another key cellular pathway: mTOR. This pathway is established as important in the regulation of multiple oncologic processes, such as cell survival and angiogenesis. mTOR is a serine/threonine kinase involved in cell response to energy depletion and hypoxia. mTOR

up-regulation is implicated in both chemotherapy and radiotherapy resistance.[9] Through immunohistochemical analysis, mTOR has been found up-regulated in RCC compared with normal renal tissue.[10] After binding of VEGF, PDGF, or other growth factors to a receptor tyrosine kinase, phosphatidylinositol 3-kinase (PI3K) is activated. Protein kinase B (Akt) is recruited and able to activate mTOR. mTOR can also be activated Akt by phosphorylation. Akt can then inhibit cell apoptosis by inactivating proteins, such as procaspase-9 and AKD1.[8] mTOR is also able to activate ribosomal protein S6 kinase, which has broad effects on cell physiology and survival. Increased S6 kinase expression is associated with more aggressive RCC.[11]

OVERVIEW OF TREATMENTS OF mRCC
Surgery

Despite mRCC being a systemic disease, surgery continues to play a role in its optimal treatment. Traditionally, this role was reserved for palliation in patients with symptoms of pain or bleeding. Given the lack of effective systemic therapy, many patients underwent cytoreductive nephrectomy (CN) with the presumption that removing a large portion of the tumor burden would improve response to systemic therapy. Although rare, spontaneous regression of metastases was seen after CN, indicating a beneficial biologic response to the surgery. There are hypotheses for CN improving

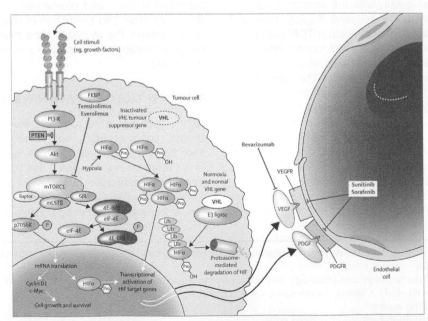

Fig. 1. Biologic pathways and therapeutic targets in RCC. (*Reprinted from* Rini BI, Campbell SC, Escudier B. Renal cell carcinoma. Lancet 2009;373:1119–32; with permission from Elsevier.)

survival, the most prominent that the primary tumor suppresses the activation of T cells.[12] By removing this suppression, the immune system has greater activity against sites of metastasis. Another possible mechanism is the beneficial removal of cells that produce tumor-related growth factors that result in abnormal signaling pathways.

Early experience with CN showed that morbidity from surgery precluded many patients from receiving immunotherapy. One study found that in patients with an Eastern Cooperative Oncology Group (ECOG) performance status ranging from 0 to 2, only 23% were able to undergo immunotherapy after CN.[13] This pattern of treatment called into question the benefit of CN. Since then, however, 2 randomized trials have examined the survival after CN plus interferon-α versus interferon-α alone. The Southwest Oncology Group (SWOG) trial, which included 120 patients from 1991 to 1998, found that CN was associated with a statistically significant 3-month survival advantage (11.1 vs 8.1 months).[14,15] The European Organisation for Research and Treatment of Cancer (EORTC) study, which randomized 85 patients from 1995 and 1998, reported a median survival benefit of 10 months associated with CN (17 vs 7 months).[16] A combined analysis of the 2 trials found CN was associated with a 6-month median survival benefit (13.6 vs 7.8 months).[17]

There are no randomized data that demonstrate a survival benefit for CN with systemic targeted therapy. Thus, many have extrapolated the benefit of CN from the experience with immunotherapy to targeted drugs. Another argument for CN's role in the era of targeted therapy is that the study population for targeted therapy included mainly those who have had a prior nephrectomy. Because the vast majority of patients enrolled in these studies had undergone nephrectomy, it is difficult to translate the positive findings of the phase 3 trials to patients who do not undergo CN.[18]

Metastatectomy for RCC was described in 1939 in a patient who lived 23 years after surgery, ultimately dying of coronary artery disease.[19,20] In the absence of effective systemic therapy, metastatectomy was thought a reasonable approach to controlling systemic disease in select patients. Multiple studies have demonstrated favorable survival in select patients after judicious metastasectomy, with 5-year survival rates ranging from 35% to 60%.[12] There are important caveats, however, to metastasectomy. First, it is unclear to what extent indolent cancer biology contributed to improved survival. Also, the role of metastatectomy in the targeted therapy era has yet to be clearly defined. Lastly, there are currently no prospective or randomized data that can

accurately determine the survival impact of metastasectomy. Despite these limitations, metastatectomy remains a viable option in highly selected patients with mRCC.

Systemic Therapy

Immunotherapy was a standard systemic treatment of mRCC in the 1980s. Cytokine therapy remains the only treatment that offers a chance of achieving a durable complete response. The cytokines interferon-α and interleukin (IL)-2 are generally associated with low rates of response and high levels of toxicity. Interferon-α has a complete response rate of 2.5% and a partial response rate of 26%.[21,22] IL-2 has a complete response rate of approximately 5% to 7% and a 15% to 20% overall response rate.[23] In the past, high-dose IL-2 has been associated with treatment mortality as high as 4%. Better patient selection and supportive care have helped mitigate many of these toxicities.

Unlike immunotherapy, targeted therapy theoretically offers more specific sites of action and less toxicity (see **Fig. 1**). Tyrosine kinase inhibitors that target angiogenesis pathways include sunitinib, sorafenib, pazopanib, tivozanib, and axitinib, which are shown to improve either overall survival (OS) or progression-free survival (PFS) in various mRCC patient contexts.

In a randomized phase 3 study, sunitinib improved PFS compared with interferon-α in treatment-naïve patients (11 vs 5 months).[24] Sorafenib as first-line therapy was found to have similar PFS compared with interferon-α in a phase 2 study. Sorafenib, however, had superior tumor control compared with interferon-α as well as a benefit in PFS in those who underwent dose escalation or crossover from interferon-α.[25] Sorafenib as a second-line therapy has been shown to significantly improve PFS compared with placebo (5.5 vs 2.8 months).[26] Pazopanib has been shown to improve PFS in treatment-naïve and immunotherapy-treated patients compared with placebo in a phase 3 trial (9.2 vs 4.2 months).[27] Axitinib, a second-generation tyrosine kinase inhibitor with more potent VEGF inhibition, has been evaluated as a second-line treatment of mRCC with a recent randomized study reporting longer PFS compared with sorafenib (6.7 vs 4.7 months).[28] Most recently, tivozanib was reported to improve PFS compared with sorafenib in the frontline setting.[29]

There are several tyrosine kinases that remain in development. Dovitinib inhibits multiple receptors, including fibroblast growth factor receptor, which is implicated as an escape mechanism after

VEGF-targeted therapy.[30] Erlotinib is an inhibitor of the epidermal growth factor receptor, which has had a response rate of 11% in metastatic papillary RCC in a phase 2 trial.[31] A follow-up trial of erlotinib plus the c-MET inhibitor ARQ 197 is in development by SWOG for advanced papillary RCC.

Another type of therapy targeting the VEGF receptor is bevacizumab, a monoclonal antibody against VEGF. One randomized, double-blind, phase 3 trial compared bevacizumab plus interferon-α to interferon-α plus placebo in treatment-naïve patients. This study reported that bevacizumab plus interferon-α significantly improved PFS compared with the control group (10.2 vs 5.4 months).[32] Later analysis showed a numerically higher median OS with bevacizumab (23.3 vs 21.3 months), but this did not reach significance ($P = .129$).[33] A similar randomized phase 3 trial compared bevacizumab plus interferon-α to interferon-α monotherapy, again failing to find a significant improvement in OS with bevacizumab (18.3 vs 17.4 months, $P = .97$) but showing a higher response rate and improved PFS for the bevacizumab arm.[34]

Temsirolimus and everolimus act by inhibiting mTOR and were Food and Drug Administration approved for the treatment of mRCC after the results of large phase 3 registration studies. Temsirolimus was evaluated in a multicenter, phase 3, randomized trial of temsirolimus versus interferon-α versus temsirolimus plus interferon-α in treatment-naïve, poor-risk patients that included 20% with non–clear cell histology. The trial reported that temsirolimus significantly improved PFS (5.5 vs 3.1 months) and OS (10.9 vs 7.3 months) compared with interferon-α.[35] Everolimus was tested in a randomized, double-blind, placebo-controlled crossover trial as second-line therapy in patients who had progressed on tyrosine kinase inhibitors of VEGF receptor, such as sunitinib and/or sorafenib. Everolimus was shown to significantly prolong PFS (4.0 vs 1.9 months).[36]

PROGNOSTICATION
Clinical Biomarkers

Risk stratification has emerged as an important clinical instrument useful in patient counseling, designing of clinical trials, and selecting appropriate therapies. Use of clinical markers for risk stratifications takes a broad view of a tumor's biology and also takes into account individual response to the tumor. The most widely used risk criteria for mRCC were developed by Motzer and colleagues[37] at the Memorial Sloan-Kettering Cancer Center (MSKCC). Five risk factors were identified as most prognostic in survival: low

performance status, high lactate dehydrogenase, low serum hemoglobin, high corrected serum calcium, and time from initial RCC diagnosis to start of systemic therapy of less than 1 year. Patients with none of these risk factors are categorized as favorable risk, those with 1 or 2 risk factors have intermediate-risk disease, and those with 3 or more risk factors are categorized as poor risk. In a study examining these criteria in patients undergoing treatment with interferon-α, median survival was 30 months in the favorable-risk group, 14 months in the intermediate-risk group, and 5 months in the poor-risk group.

The MSKCC criteria have been externally validated and additional predictors of survival elucidated.[38] A study of treatment-naïve patients with mRCC enrolled in clinical trials found prior radiotherapy and the presence of liver, lung, and retroperitoneal nodal metastases as independent predictors of survival.[38] The other notable clinical prognostic criteria, the University of California Los Angeles Integrated Staging System, uses TNM staging, ECOG performance status, and Fuhrman grade. This system has also been validated and is associated with survival.[39]

Prognostic factors for OS in patients treated with VEGF-targeted therapy were examined by Heng and colleagues[40] in a study of 645 patients treated with VEGF therapy for the first time. There was agreement with 4 MSKCC criteria associated with worse survival: anemia, hypercalcemia, Karnofsky performance scale status (KPS) less than 80%, and time from diagnosis to treatment of less than 1 year. In addition, neutrophilia and thrombocytosis were identified as adverse prognostic factors. Of these 6 factors, patients were divided into risk categories: favorable (no prognostic factors), intermediate (1–2 prognostic factors), and poor (3–6 prognostic factors). Two-year OS rates for the groups were 75%, 53%, and 7%, respectively.

A similar study examined prognostic factors in patients with clear cell RCC (ccRCC) undergoing treatment with bevacizumab, sorafenib, sunitinib, or axitinib. Five factors were found associated with worse PFS on multivariate analysis: time from diagnosis to treatment of less than 2 years, baseline platelet count greater than 300 K/μL, baseline neutrophil count greater than 4.5 K/μL, corrected serum calcium less than 8.5 mg/dL or greater than 10 mg/dL, and initial ECOG performance status greater than 0. Using these clinical factors, 3 prognostic groups were formed with a median PFS that was 20 months in the favorable-risk group (0–1 factor), 13 months in the intermediate-risk group (2 factors), and 3.9 months in the poor-risk group (>2 factors).[41]

Molecular Biomarkers

An emerging method of prognostication is with molecular biomarkers. These markers can be used to determine prognosis independently and can add to the accuracy of current prognostic models. **Table 1** provides a summary of the many molecular markers in RCC and their association with various outcomes.[42]

A carbonic anhydrase enzyme, CAIX is one of the more notable markers given its specificity for RCC. It has not been identified in healthy renal tissue and is expressed in almost all cases of ccRCC.[43] CAIX is involved in the reversible reaction that converts water and carbon dioxide to bicarbonate and a hydrogen cation. Increased levels of CAIX are necessary for pH balance in a tumor's microenvironment of hypoxia and acidosis.[44] Using immunohistochemistry and a threshold of 85% CAIX staining, Bui and colleagues[45] found that lower CAIX levels were independently associated with poor survival in patients with advanced RCC. The reason for this association is not entirely clear, although the authors hypothesize that CAIX may be more important in the early stages of tumorigenesis to deal with hypoxia. Therefore, CAIX may not be as important in mRCC, which can account for the observed low levels of expression. Another study of patients with ccRCC found that low CAIX expression was associated with worsened survival, although it was not an independent predictor when adjusting for other factors, such as nuclear grade.[43]

VEGF levels within the tumor can also be used as a prognostic marker. Opposite from CAIX, increased expression in tissue samples has been shown to predict worse survival.[46] The combination of low expression of CAIX and high expression of VEGF was shown more accurate in prognostication than when evaluating these markers individually. Serum VEGF may also have a role in prognostication of mRCC, because these levels correlate well with tissue levels of VEGF.[47] Jacobsen and colleagues[48] examined serum VEGF before surgery and found increases associated with decreased survival. In mRCC, elevated serum VEGF has been correlated with decreased survival; however, VEGF levels were not independently prognostic on multivariate analysis.[49]

HIF-1α has been studied as a marker for ccRCC because its expression is significantly elevated compared with benign renal tissue. Its increased nuclear expression has been shown a predictor of worse survival in metastatic disease (13.5 vs 24.4 months) on multivariate analysis.[50] Other investigators examining cytoplasmic levels of HIF-1α, however, found high expression was associated with significantly longer survival.[51] HIF-1α levels were not associated with survival in patients with non–clear cell histology or those categorized as poor risk.[51,52] Further research into the role of HIF-1α, including emerging evidence that it has a role as a tumor suppressor, can help explain these reported differences.[53]

A panel of molecular markers has been found an independent predictor of poor outcome in patients with ccRCC.[54] The expression of B7-H1, survivin, and Ki-67 together formed a BioScore that is able to predicted RCC-specific death on multivariate analysis. Kim and colleagues[55] examined tissue from 150 patients with metastatic ccRCC with tissue array examining expression of CAIX, phosphatase and tensin homolog (PTEN), vimentin, and protein 53 (p53). Using these markers, they were able to predict disease-specific survival on multivariate analysis. The corrected concordance index of this tissue array was superior to the University of California Los Angeles Integrated Staging System. When this group examined tissue from both localized and mRCC, they found the combination of clinical and molecular factors was a more prognostic than the either one independently.[56]

PREDICTING RESPONSE TO SYSTEMIC THERAPY

The previous section describes the many biomarkers that can assist in prognostication, which provide information about the cancer outcome independent of the treatment administered. Predictive markers, alternatively, give information on disease outcome based on a specific treatment. Many prognostic markers have been examined for their predictive potential. Predictive markers better identify responders or nonresponders to different therapies, allowing for more personalized care. Currently, there are no validated biomarkers that predict response to systemic therapy. The next section reviews pathologic, clinical, molecular, and genetic markers that have shown promise in predicting response.

Immunotherapy

Patients with certain pathologic features respond better to IL-2. IL-2 has been shown more effective in ccRCC with alveolar features, no papillary features, and no granular features.[57] A study examining CAIX expression in pathology specimens in patients receiving IL-2 found an increased level of CAIX predicted improved survival.[58] Those with high expression of CAIX were 3.3 times more likely to respond to high-dose IL-2 compared with those with low expression.[59] A prospective trial is

Table 1
Molecular markers and their associations with prognosis, progression-free survival, overall survival, cancer-specific mortality, treatment efficacy, and added value in established risk stratification for renal cell carcinoma

Marker	Prognosis	PFS	OS	CSM	Treatment Efficacy	Added Value in Prognostic Models
Neutrophil		+	+ (In IL-2 patients)	+	NS (low response rate in IL-2 patients)	+ (Leibovich)
C-reactive protein			+			+
VHL		+/NS	+/NS	+	+ (Predicts response to targeted therapy)	+
HIF-α			+		+ (Predicts response to sunitinib)	
Tissue based						
VEGF	+	+		+		
CAIX	+					+
mTOR						
pS6			+		+ (Predicts response to temsirolimus)	
PTEN			+		+ (Predicts response to mTOR inhibitors)/ns (low response in temsirolimus)	
pAkt	+ (For localized and mRCC)			+	+ (Predicts response to temsirolimus)	
Other						
Caveolin-1			+/NS (coexpression with Akt/mTOR)			

Marker			
p53		NS	
Ki-67	+	+	+ (Coexpression with CAIX)
Survivin	+	+	
B7-H1	+	+	+
Vimentin		+	
Fascin	+		
MMP		+	
IMP3	+	+	+ (SSIGN)
Blood based			
VEGF	+/NS	+/NS (in mRCC)/+ (in sorafenib patients)	+ (Predicts response rate in sunitinib)/ns (does not predict response rate in sorafenib)
CAIX	+	+	
NGAL	+	+	
SAA	+		
IGF-I	+		
NMP-22			

Abbreviations: CSM, cancer-specific mortality; IGF-I, insulin-like growth factor; IMP3, insulin-like growth factor II mRNA-binding protein; MMP, matrix metalloproteinases; NGAL, neutrophil gelatinase–associated lipocalin; NMP-22, nuclear matrix protein–22; NS, not significant; +, association; SAA, serum amyloid A.

Reprinted from Sun M, Shariat SF, Cheng C, et al. Prognostic factors and predictive models in renal cell carcinoma: a contemporary review. Eur Urol 2011;60:644–61; with permission from Elsevier.

currently under way examining administration of high-dose IL-2 using a model that includes CAIX expression. Preliminary results, however, have not shown any pretreatment clinical factors to predict response.[60]

The gene that encodes for CAIX protein is *CA9*, which is a potential predictive marker for mRCC. The gene has known single nucleotide polymorphisms (SNPs), which are common in patients with ccRCC. Certain SNPs are associated with improved OS and likelihood of response to IL-2.[61] Further studies are necessary to determine if *CA9* and CAIX can be used to predict which patients respond to IL-2.

VEGF-Targeted Therapy

Treatment-associated hypertension has been investigated as an important clinical marker for evaluating the efficacy of therapy targeting VEGF. Hypertension is a known side effect of angiogenesis inhibitors, such that uncontrolled hypertension is a relative contraindication to their use. In the phase 3 trial of sunitinib, the incidence of hypertension was 24%.[24] Because VEGF stimulates nitric oxide and prostacyclin production, it acts by inhibiting vasodilatory mechanisms. Targeting VEGF, therefore, leads to a net increase in peripheral vascular resistance.

A retrospective analysis of patients treated with sunitinib examined blood pressure (BP) on days 1 and 28 of treatment. Patients with sunitinib-induced hypertension had significantly improved PFS (12.5 vs 2.5 months) and OS (30.9 vs 7.2 months) compared with those without hypertension.[62] There was no significant increase in hypertension-associated adverse events. Diastolic hypertension was evaluated during treatment with axitinib in phase 2 studies of various solid tumors, including RCC. Patients with a diastolic BP greater than or equal to 90 mm Hg during treatment had a significantly lower risk of death (hazard ratio [HR] 0.55) and higher objective response rate (44% vs 12%). The rate of progression was also lower in those with a higher diastolic BP (HR 0.76), although it was not statistically significant.[63] BP and its association with survival were also evaluated in the randomized trial of bevacizumab plus interferon-α.[34] The study showed that treatment-induced hypertension significantly improvement in PFS (13.2 vs 8 months) and OS (41.6 vs 16.2 months). Development of hypertension after 2 months of treatment was an independent predictor of OS. These studies provide insight into the importance of host response to VEGF therapy. Hypertension may emerge as an important clinical marker for following response

to therapy and in selecting patients likely to benefit from the treatments targeting VEGF. A trial of dose titration of axitinib based on BP is ongoing.[64]

Besides clinical markers, there are several molecular and genetic markers that are promising in predicting response to systemic therapy (see **Table 1**). The *VHL* gene mutation was evaluated as predictive of survival in patients who received therapy targeting VEGF.[65] Patients with *VHL* mutation or promoter alteration had a response rate of 48% compared with 35% in those with intact *VHL*. Those with abnormal *VHL* had a longer time to progression compared with patients without *VHL* mutation (13.3 vs 7.4 months). Another study found no association between response rates after VEGF therapy in those with inactivated *VHL* mutation compared with wild-type *VHL*.[66] When examining only patients with a loss of function mutation, however, they found it was associated with a significantly better response rate compared with wild type (52% vs 31%). Validation is required before the clinical utilization of *VHL* to predict response to VEGF therapy.

Overexpression of HIF-1α and HIF-2α levels in tissue samples has been investigated as predictive of response to VEGF targeted therapy. One study demonstrated an improved response to sunitinib in patients with ccRCC and overexpression of HIF.[67] Studies on VEGF levels as a predictive marker are mixed. One study showed that decreased serum VEGF levels predict response to sunitinib.[68] The change from baseline with sunitinib was another important predictor with larger changes in VEGF associated with improved response. In patients who progress after bevacizumab, lower baseline levels of VEGF were associated with improved PFS and response rates after sunitinib.[69] When examining VEGF levels with sorafenib treatment, they were not found predictive of response rates or survival.[70]

A study examined survival in patients treated with tyrosine kinase inhibitor and found it positively associated with levels of circulating cells, plasma angiogenic factors, and bone marrow–derived cells that migrate to sites of tumor neovascularization.[71] Lower baseline levels of CD45(dim)CD34(+) VEGFR2(+) bone marrow–derived cells were associated with improved PFS and OS. In addition, large changes in the levels of VEGF and stromal cell–derived factor-1α, a proangiogenic factor, within the first 2 weeks of treatment were associated with improved OS. These circulating biomarkers require further investigation to determine their predictive potential.

SNPs in genes, such as the VEGF receptor and PDGF receptor, have been examined prospectively in patients treated with sunitinib. In a study of 101 previously untreated patients, associations between gene SNPs were examined with respect to efficacy and toxicity with sunitinib.[72] Two missense polymorphisms in the VEGF receptor (VEGFR3) were associated with decreased PFS on multivariable analysis. VEGFR3 has expression in tumor blood vessels and is a key mediator of other proangiogenic factors. In addition to predicting survival, the CYP3A5*1 allele was associated with increased toxicity because it is involved in sunitinib metabolism. Toxicity to sunitinib is often manageable but can lead to significant delays in treatment, dose reductions, or dose suspension.[24]

mTOR Inhibitors

Increased expression of phosphorylated-S6 and phosphorylated-Akt, which are both upstream and downstream of mTOR in the signaling pathway, are associated with tumor response to temsirolimus.[73] Cho and colleagues examined 20 specimens and found no tumors with objective response to temsirolimus had low expression of these proteins. The investigators found no association between CAIX or *VHL* status with response to temsirolimus.

PTEN is a tumor suppressor protein upstream of mTOR that inhibits Akt phosphorylation. In vitro and in vivo studies have shown temsirolimus more efficacious in cells with the loss of the *PTEN* tumor suppressor gene.[74] Studies with immunohistochemical analysis have shown that tumors with lower expression of PTEN are typically more aggressive and associated with a shorter cancer-specific survival.[75] PTEN levels were not found to correlate with survival in patients treated with temsirolimus.[52]

These clinical, molecular, and genetic markers are promising in their ability to predict response to therapy. Validation of these markers is necessary. Ultimately, prospective studies using these markers in a pretreatment algorithm can move treatment for mRCC to an even more individualized approach.

TREATMENT PARADIGM BASED ON INDIVIDUALIZED FACTORS

mRCC is a complex disease with multiple treatment options and stages of presentation. This discussion assists in developing a treatment paradigm for mRCC based on individual clinical factors. **Figs. 2–4** provide algorithms for selecting treatments in patients with mRCC with a primary tumor, systemic treatment naïve, and failed first-line therapy. These figures use data from the International Consultation on Urological Diseases and the European Association of Urology guidelines on mRCC.[76]

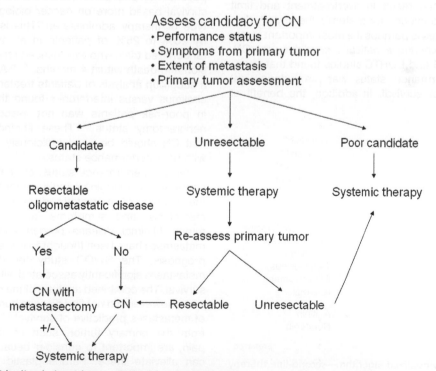

Fig. 2. Individualized algorithm—mRCC with primary tumor.

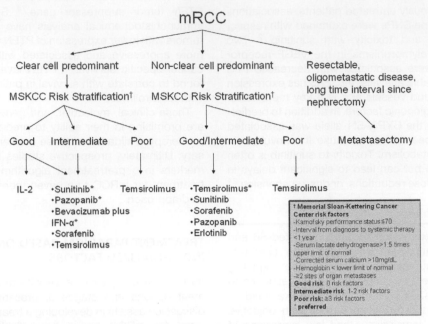

Fig. 3. Individualized algorithm—systemic treatment-naïve mRCC.

Patient Selection for Cytoreductive Nephrectomy

Although randomized studies have demonstrated an OS benefit with CN, not all patients with mRCC benefit from the surgery. Poor patient selection can result in overtreatment and limit patients' candidacy for systemic therapy. Performance status is perhaps the most important factor when considering a patient's candidacy for CN. The SWOG and EORTC studies found that favorable performance status was an independent predictor of survival. In addition, the benefit of

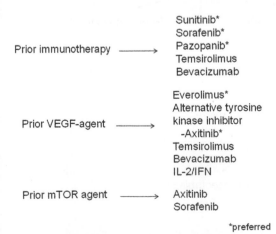

Fig. 4. Individualized algorithm—second-line therapy for mRCC.

CN was seen in both patients with an ECOG performance status of 0 or 1. Because the studies did not include those with a performance status of 2 or 3, it is not clear if this population receives the same benefit from CN. It is generally regarded that patients with poor performance status have limited survival based more on cancer biology than the type of therapy administered. This is illustrated by 20% to 25% of patients in all arms of the randomized trials who experienced rapid progression and death within 4 months.[14,16] Additionally, a subgroup analysis of patients treated with temsirolimus versus interferon-α found that survival in poor-risk patients was not associated with nephrectomy status.[77] These findings indicate that CN should be used judiciously in patients with poor performance status.

Besides performance status, clinical factors to consider when judging candidacy for CN include the amount of metastatic disease, organs of metastasis, and symptoms from the primary tumor. Minimal disease burden and lung-only metastases have been thought to portend a better prognosis. The SWOG study found lung-only metastases significantly associated with improved survival. The combined analysis of the randomized trials, however, did not find disease burden or sites of metastases predictive of survival.[17] Symptoms from the primary tumor, such as bleeding or pain, are important to consider because surgery can alleviate these. Paraneoplastic syndromes can be treated with nephrectomy, though it is

		Nephrectomy: Immunotherapy planned		Nephrectomy: Targeted therapy planned	
		Metastatic burden		Metastatic burden	
		Limited	Extensive	Limited	Extensive
Good surgical risk	With symptoms related to primary tumor	Appropriate		Appropriate	
	Without symptoms related to primary tumor			Uncertain	Uncertain
Poor surgical risk	With symptoms related to primary tumor	Uncertain			
	Without symptoms related to primary tumor			Inappropriate	

Fig. 5. Appropriateness ratings are shown for CN in patients with mRCC with primary tumor in situ who did not receive prior immunotherapy. The boxes are labeled as an appropriate rating, uncertain rating (disagreement among panelists) and inappropriate rating. (*Reprinted from* Halbert RJ, Figlin RA, Atkins MB, et al. Treatment of patients with metastatic renal cell cancer: a RAND Appropriateness Panel. Cancer 2006;107(10):2375–83; with permission from John Wiley and Sons.)

unclear with CN without metastatectomy is effective in mRCC.

Given the often difficult decision of selecting patients for CN, consensus opinions have been drawn from medical oncologists and urologists regarding its appropriateness.[78] After an extensive literature review, an expert panel rated CN as appropriate, uncertain, and inappropriate in different clinical settings (**Fig. 5**). In patients with good surgical risk, symptoms related to the primary tumor and limited metastatic burden, the panel thought that CN is appropriate if targeted therapy is planned. If immunotherapy is planned, the appropriateness of CN is extended to symptomatic patients with extensive metastasis or asymptomatic patients with limited disease. In patients who are poor surgical risk and asymptomatic from the primary tumor, CN is thought inappropriate in most cases. In the other clinical permutations, including those with extensive metastatic disease, the role of CN is unclear.

Timing of Cytoreductive Nephrectomy

The knowledge that a subset of patients experiences rapid progression despite surgery has led to the use of up-front systemic therapy to determine patients who will benefit from CN. Bex and colleagues[79] examined 16 patients with mRCC treated initially with 2 courses of IL-2 and interferon-α. Five of the patients progressed and were not offered surgery. The remaining underwent CN followed by additional immunotherapy with a mean OS of 11.5 months; the results are comparable to the survival in the CN arms in the SWOG and EORTC trials. This demonstrated that immunotherapy may safely be used to select the subset of patients unlikely to benefit from surgery, saving them the morbidity of surgery.

The use of targeted molecular therapy in a neoadjuvant manner is more attractive than immunotherapy given its better efficacy and lower toxicity. One prospective study examined intermediate-risk and poor-risk patients treated with sunitinib for 12 to 16 weeks before CN[80]; 29% did not ultimately undergo CN, mostly due to disease progression. The OS for the group was 15.2 months (26 months for intermediate-risk disease and 9 months for poor-risk disease), which compares favorably with the randomized phase 3 trial comparing sunitinib with interferon-α (21 months for intermediate-risk disease and 5.3 months for poor-risk disease). There are currently 4 ongoing clinical trials examining neoadjuvant sunitinib or sorafenib followed by CN. Other randomized trials examine sorafenib or sunitinib given after CN.[12] The results of these studies will better delineate the role of CN in mRCC.[81]

Another benefit of targeted therapy is the potential for reduction of primary tumor volume, which can be useful in patients with tumors too large for resection. One study examined 19 patients with advanced RCC who had a primary tumor that was unresectable at the time of presentation. After 4 weeks of sunitinib, 16% of patients had partial response of the primary tumor that facilitated future CN.[82] Additionally, there is a report of RCC with tumor thrombus that was downstaged with sunitinib before resection.[83] In general, however, molecular therapies have little effect on tumor thrombi. In a study of 25 patients with RCC with tumor thrombus, 44% had a decrease in thrombus after targeted therapy although only 12% had such a response that it changed thrombus classification.[84] Primary tumor response after neoadjuvant therapy has not been overwhelming, although it can convert select patients into operative candidates. There are concerns with regards to the safety of neoadjuvant therapy because inhibition of angiogenesis may have unwanted postoperative effects. Studies examining surgical complication rates, however, have not shown rates of delayed wound healing or dehiscence to be significantly increased.[85,86]

Patient Selection for Metastatectomy

The main factor that portends favorable outcomes after metastasectomy is a disease-free interval greater than 12 months from treatment of the primary tumor to metastasis. Other important factors are the number of metastases, the ability of complete resection, and the sites of metastases. The importance of complete resection is shown in a restrospective study of 887 patients.[87] All patients had multiple sites of metastasis and 14% were able to undergo complete surgical resection of all metastases. Complete resection was associated with a longer cancer-specific survival (4.8 vs 1.3 years) and was particularly beneficial in patients with lung-only metastases. Patients with multiple metastases involving organs other than the lung still benefited from complete resection. Additionally, the benefit of metastasectomy was seen for both synchronous and metachronous metastases.

A study by Kavolius and colleagues[88] reported lung metastases, solitary metastases, and age less than 60 independently predictive of improved survival with metastasectomy. Another study found favorable-risk stratification by MSKCC criteria and undergoing metastatectomy independently associated with improved survival.[89] Metastasectomy was found beneficial to patients in all risk categories.

Patient Selection for Immunotherapy

IL-2 and interferon-α, although largely supplanted by targeted therapy as first-line therapy, still have a role in the treatment of mRCC. As discussed previously, these therapies offer a small chance of cure, which is not seen with targeted therapy. Therefore, in patients with no MSKCC adverse risk factors and good organ function, high-dose IL-2 is an option for first-line therapy. In the studies of IL-2, ECOG performance status was found predictive of response.[23] IL-2 may have a role as second-line treatment after VEGF-targeted therapies. Interferon-α can be used in conjunction with bevacizumab as both first- and second-line therapy.

Patient Selection for Targeted First-Line Therapy

Accompanying the influx of new targeted treatment options are many questions regarding patient selection. Key factors in determining optimal first-line treatment include histology and risk stratification. Most studies using targeted therapy included only patients with predominant clear cell histology. The randomized phase 3 trials of sunitinib, sorafenib, pazopanib, and bevacizumab plus interferon included only patients with ccRCC. Despite the lack of randomized data on the use of sunitinib in non-ccRCC, there are data that demonstrate its use in more varied conditions. An expanded access study included patients with poor performance status and non-ccRCC, demonstrating sunitinib was both safe and efficacious in this population.[90] The objective response rate for patients was 11% compared with 17% for the entire group.

As opposed to tyrosine kinase inhibitors, which have limited efficacy in non–clear cell histology, the mTOR inhibitor temsirolimus has shown better effectiveness. A subgroup analysis of the phase 3 trial of temsirolimus found the OS in patients with non-ccRCC was 11.6 months compared with 4.3 months in those treated with interferon-α.[91] Temsirolimus had a much smaller benefit in patients with clear cell histology (10.7 vs 8.2 months). Therefore, temsirolimus is the first-line systemic therapy of choice in non–clear cell histology RCC.

Risk stratification's importance in selecting systemic therapy derives from the use of performance status and other MSKCC criteria to determine inclusion and exclusion in clinical trials. For example, 90% of the population treated in the randomized phase 3 trial of sunitinib versus interferon-α were good risk or intermediate risk.[24] The sorafenib trial did not include poor-risk patients.[70] The randomized trials of bevacizumab plus interferon-α and of pazopanib only included patients with more favorable performance status (ECOG 0–1 or KPS ≥70).[27,34] There are few randomized data examining the efficacy of therapies targeting VEGF in poor-risk patients. The expanded access trial, discussed previously, demonstrated a 9% objective response rate in patients with ECOG score of greater than or equal to 2.[90]

In good-risk and intermediate-risk patients with predominantly clear cell histology who are not candidates for IL-2, there are 3 preferred treatment options. These include sunitinib, pazopanib, and bevacizumab plus interferon-α, all shown to improve PFS. Sorafenib did not show an improvement in PFS compared with interferon-α in its phase 3 trial.[70]

The randomized trial that included mainly poor-risk patients involved temsirolimus. The study included 82% of patients with a KPS less than or equal to 70 and 74% of patients categorized as poor risk by MSKCC criteria.[35] In the study, temsirolimus improved OS by 3.6 months compared with interferon-α. Therefore, temsirolimus is the treatment of choice in poor-risk patients.

There are additional clinical factors to consider besides histology and those used by MSKCC criteria. Utility of targeted therapy is unclear in patients with CNS metastases because these patients were typically excluded from the clinical trials. The trial to include patients with CNS metastases was temsirolimus, although patients were required to have stable disease and not have had corticosteroids after surgery or radiotherapy.[35] The trial examining broader utilization of sunitinib with expanded criteria found a 12% objective response rate in patients with brain metastases.[90]

Those with organ dysfunction may not be the best candidates for targeted therapy. All the clinical trials, including the temsirolimus study, excluded those without adequate renal, hepatic, hematologic, and cardiac function. Those with a recent cardiovascular event were also excluded. Lastly, uncontrolled hypertension is a concern for therapies targeting VEGF, because treatment-associated hypertension can be an adverse event. Those with a systolic BP greater than or equal to140 to 160 and diastolic BP greater than or equal to 90 mm Hg on antihypertensive mediation were excluded from the phase 3 randomized trials. Use of targeted therapy in patients with these poor clinical features should be done with caution.

Patient Selection for Second-Line Therapy

Attempts at combined therapy have been largely unsuccessful due to high levels of toxicity, which has brought the focus of attention to sequential therapy. When selecting second-line therapy, prior systemic therapy is the most important factor. Thus far, only everolimus and axitinib have demonstrated improvement in PFS after failed VEGF therapy.[28,36] A study of sorafenib administration in sunitinib-refractory patients found only 10% of patients had a partial response.[92] In patients who have progressed despite immunotherapy, sorafenib, pazopanib, and axitinib have shown improved PFS. Of these, axitinib is associated with improved PFS compared with sorafenib.[28] Data on therapy after mTOR first-line treatment are limited. Twenty-four patients who failed temsirolimus were treated with axitinib and sorafenib. Longer PFS was seen in those randomized to axitinib, although this was not statistically significant.[28]

There are few data examining patient factors that may help with selecting appropriate second-line therapy. Patient factors and the characteristics of first-line treatment, such as duration of treatment or degree of response, require further investigation to determine if they influence response to second-line treatment.

FUTURE OF INDIVIDUALIZED THERAPY

As the biology of mRCC is better understood, identifying patients based mainly on histology can be shifted to focusing on their cancer biology at a cellular level. This individualized care holds the promise of treating specific aberrant molecular pathways involved in tumorigenesis. In the process of individualizing care at a molecular level, an extremely complex system involving the tumor, the host, and the therapy has been uncovered. All 3 of these factors are interconnected and their dynamic relationship is only beginning to be understood. Further research focusing on this interplay is necessary to identify better predictors of response, new targets for therapy, and a molecular basis for sequential therapy.

SUMMARY

Treatment of mRCC has changed dramatically and is moving toward a more individualized strategy. This strategy relies on multiple factors for prognostication and prediction of response that include clinical, genetic, pathologic, and molecular markers. Great strides have been made in identifying types of therapies that have good efficacy in certain subsets of patients. A validated marker that accurately predicts treatment failure or success, however, is still lacking. Further research to elucidate the molecular changes of mRCC induced by treatment and the host is necessary.

- mRCC exhibits tremendous genetic, biologic, and clinical diversity.
- The goal of individualized care can make treatment more efficacious while limiting morbidity.
- Better understanding of molecular pathways can lead to diagnosing the key aberrant pathways in patients with mRCC.
- There is an abundance of biomarkers that help in prognostication and may soon predict response to treatment.
- Currently there are no validated markers that can accurately predict treatment success or failure.
- An individualized treatment strategy of mRCC is approaching, although further research is required to validate biomarkers and further elucidate the molecular changes induced by treatment and the host immune response.

REFERENCES

1. Bukowski RM. Natural history and therapy of metastatic renal cell carcinoma: the role of interleukin-2. Cancer 1997;80(7):1198–220.

2. Vaupel P, Mayer A. Hypoxia in cancer: significance and impact on clinical outcome. Cancer Metastasis Rev 2007;26(2):225–39.

3. Rini BI, Campbell SC, Escudier B. Renal cell carcinoma. Lancet 2009;373(9669):1119–32.

4. Duan DR, Pause A, Burgess WH, et al. Inhibition of transcription elongation by the VHL tumor suppressor protein. Science 1995;269(5229):1402–6.

5. Kibel A, Iliopoulos O, DeCaprio JA, et al. Binding of the von Hippel-Lindau tumor suppressor protein to Elongin B and C. Science 1995;269(5229):1444–6.

6. Pause A, Lee S, Worrell RA, et al. The von Hippel-Lindau tumor-suppressor gene product forms a stable complex with human CUL-2, a member of the Cdc53 family of proteins. Proc Natl Acad Sci U S A 1997;94(6):2156–61.

7. Kaelin WG Jr. The von Hippel-Lindau gene, kidney cancer, and oxygen sensing. J Am Soc Nephrol 2003;14(11):2703–11.

8. Banumathy G, Cairns P. Signaling pathways in renal cell carcinoma. Cancer Biol Ther 2010;10(7): 658–64.

9. Hudes GR. Targeting mTOR in renal cell carcinoma. Cancer 2009;115(Suppl 10):2313–20.

10. Robb VA, Karbowniczek M, Klein-Szanto AJ, et al. Activation of the mTOR signaling pathway in renal clear cell carcinoma. J Urol 2007;177(1):346–52.

11. Hager M, Haufe H, Alinger B, et al. pS6 expression in normal renal parenchyma, primary renal cell carcinomas and their metastases. Pathol Oncol Res 2011. DOI:10.1007/s12253-011-9439-y. [Epub ahead of print].

12. Russo P. Multi-modal treatment for metastatic renal cancer: the role of surgery. World J Urol 2010; 28(3):295–301.

13. Bennett RT, Lerner SE, Taub HC, et al. Cytoreductive surgery for stage IV renal cell carcinoma. J Urol 1995;154(1):32–4.

14. Flanigan RC, Salmon SE, Blumenstein BA, et al. Nephrectomy followed by interferon alfa-2b compared with interferon alfa-2b alone for metastatic renal-cell cancer. N Engl J Med 2001;345(23):1655–9.

15. Lara PN Jr, Tangen CM, Conlon SJ, et al. Predictors of survival of advanced renal cell carcinoma: long-term results from Southwest Oncology Group Trial S8949. J Urol 2009;181(2):512–6 [discussion: 516–7].

16. Mickisch GH, Garin A, van Poppel H, et al. Radical nephrectomy plus interferon-alfa-based immunotherapy compared with interferon alfa alone in metastatic renal-cell carcinoma: a randomised trial. Lancet 2001;358(9286):966–70.

17. Flanigan RC, Mickisch G, Sylvester R, et al. Cytoreductive nephrectomy in patients with metastatic renal cancer: a combined analysis. J Urol 2004; 171(3):1071–6.

18. Spiess PE, Fishman MN. Cytoreductive nephrectomy vs medical therapy as initial treatment:

a rational approach to the sequence question in metastatic renal cell carcinoma. Cancer Control 2010;17(4):269–78.

19. Barney JD, Churchill EJ. Adenocarcinoma of the kidney with metastasis to the lung: cured by nephrectomy and lobectomy. J Urol 1939;143: 269–76.

20. Wilkins EW Jr, Burke JF, Head JM. The surgical management of metastatic neoplasms in the lung. J Thorac Cardiovasc Surg 1961;42:298–309.

21. deKernion JB, Sarna G, Figlin R, et al. The treatment of renal cell carcinoma with human leukocyte alpha-interferon. J Urol 1983;130(6):1063–6.

22. Quesada JR, Swanson DA, Trindade A, et al. Renal cell carcinoma: antitumor effects of leukocyte interferon. Cancer Res 1983;43(2):940–7.

23. Fyfe G, Fisher RI, Rosenberg SA, et al. Results of treatment of 255 patients with metastatic renal cell carcinoma who received high-dose recombinant interleukin-2 therapy. J Clin Oncol 1995;13(3): 688–96.

24. Motzer RJ, Hutson TE, Tomczak P, et al. Sunitinib versus interferon alfa in metastatic renal-cell carcinoma. N Engl J Med 2007;356(2):115–24.

25. Escudier B, Szczylik C, Hutson TE, et al. Randomized phase II trial of first-line treatment with sorafenib versus interferon Alfa-2a in patients with metastatic renal cell carcinoma. J Clin Oncol 2009;27(8):1280–9.

26. Escudier B, Eisen T, Stadler WM, et al. Sorafenib in advanced clear-cell renal-cell carcinoma. N Engl J Med 2007;356(2):125–34.

27. Sternberg CN, Davis ID, Mardiak J, et al. Pazopanib in locally advanced or metastatic renal cell carcinoma: results of a randomized phase III trial. J Clin Oncol 2010;28(6):1061–8.

28. Rini BI, Escudier B, Tomczak P, et al. Comparative effectiveness of axitinib versus sorafenib in advanced renal cell carcinoma (AXIS): a randomised phase 3 trial. Lancet 2011;378(9807):1931–9.

29. AVEO and Astellas Announce Tivozanib Successfully Demonstrated Progression-Free Survival Superiority over Sorafenib in Patients with Advanced Renal Cell Cancer in Phase 3 TIVO-1 Trial. Available at: http://www.astellas.com/en/corporate/news/detail/aveo-and-astellas-announce-tiv.html. Accessed February 19, 2012.

30. Sarker D, Molife R, Evans TR, et al. A phase I pharmacokinetic and pharmacodynamic study of TKI258, an oral, multitargeted receptor tyrosine kinase inhibitor in patients with advanced solid tumors. Clin Cancer Res 2008;14(7):2075–81.

31. Gordon MS, Hussey M, Nagle RB, et al. Phase II study of erlotinib in patients with locally advanced or metastatic papillary histology renal cell cancer: SWOG S0317. J Clin Oncol 2009;27(34):5788–93.

32. Escudier B, Pluzanska A, Koralewski P, et al. Bevacizumab plus interferon alfa-2a for treatment of

metastatic renal cell carcinoma: a randomised, double-blind phase III trial. Lancet 2007;370(9605): 2103–11.

33. Escudier B, Bellmunt J, Negrier S, et al. Phase III trial of bevacizumab plus interferon alfa-2a in patients with metastatic renal cell carcinoma (AVO-REN): final analysis of overall survival. J Clin Oncol 2010;28(13):2144–50.

34. Rini BI, Halabi S, Rosenberg JE, et al. Phase III trial of bevacizumab plus interferon alfa versus interferon alfa monotherapy in patients with metastatic renal cell carcinoma: final results of CALGB 90206. J Clin Oncol 2010;28(13):2137–43.

35. Hudes G, Carducci M, Tomczak P, et al. Temsirolimus, interferon alfa, or both for advanced renal-cell carcinoma. N Engl J Med 2007;356(22):2271–81.

36. Motzer RJ, Escudier B, Oudard S, et al. Efficacy of everolimus in advanced renal cell carcinoma: a double-blind, randomised, placebo-controlled phase III trial. Lancet 2008;372(9637):449–56.

37. Motzer RJ, Bacik J, Murphy BA, et al. Interferon-alfa as a comparative treatment for clinical trials of new therapies against advanced renal cell carcinoma. J Clin Oncol 2002;20(1):289–96.

38. Mekhail TM, Abou-Jawde RM, Boumerhi G, et al. Validation and extension of the Memorial Sloan-Kettering prognostic factors model for survival in patients with previously untreated metastatic renal cell carcinoma. J Clin Oncol 2005;23(4):832–41.

39. Patard JJ, Kim HL, Lam JS, et al. Use of the University of California Los Angeles integrated staging system to predict survival in renal cell carcinoma: an international multicenter study. J Clin Oncol 2004;22(16):3316–22.

40. Heng DY, Xie W, Regan MM, et al. Prognostic factors for overall survival in patients with metastatic renal cell carcinoma treated with vascular endothelial growth factor-targeted agents: results from a large, multicenter study. J Clin Oncol 2009;27(34):5794–9.

41. Choueiri TK, Garcia JA, Elson P, et al. Clinical factors associated with outcome in patients with metastatic clear-cell renal cell carcinoma treated with vascular endothelial growth factor-targeted therapy. Cancer 2007;110(3):543–50.

42. Sun M, Shariat SF, Cheng C, et al. Prognostic factors and predictive models in renal cell carcinoma: a contemporary review. Eur Urol 2011;60(4):644–61.

43. Leibovich BC, Sheinin Y, Lohse CM, et al. Carbonic anhydrase IX is not an independent predictor of outcome for patients with clear cell renal cell carcinoma. J Clin Oncol 2007;25(30):4757–64.

44. Wykoff CC, Beasley NJ, Watson PH, et al. Hypoxia-inducible expression of tumor-associated carbonic anhydrases. Cancer Res 2000;60(24):7075–83.

45. Bui MH, Seligson D, Han KR, et al. Carbonic anhydrase IX is an independent predictor of survival in advanced renal clear cell carcinoma: implications for prognosis and therapy. Clin Cancer Res 2003; 9(2):802–11.

46. Phuoc NB, Ehara H, Gotoh T, et al. Prognostic value of the co-expression of carbonic anhydrase IX and vascular endothelial growth factor in patients with clear cell renal cell carcinoma. Oncol Rep 2008; 20(3):525–30.

47. Rioux-Leclercq N, Fergelot P, Zerrouki S, et al. Plasma level and tissue expression of vascular endothelial growth factor in renal cell carcinoma: a prospective study of 50 cases. Hum Pathol 2007; 38(10):1489–95.

48. Jacobsen J, Rasmuson T, Grankvist K, et al. Vascular endothelial growth factor as prognostic factor in renal cell carcinoma. J Urol 2000;163(1):343–7.

49. Negrier S, Perol D, Menetrier-Caux C, et al. Interleukin-6, interleukin-10, and vascular endothelial growth factor in metastatic renal cell carcinoma: prognostic value of interleukin-6–from the Groupe Francais d'Immunotherapie. J Clin Oncol 2004; 22(12):2371–8.

50. Klatte T, Seligson DB, Riggs SB, et al. Hypoxia-inducible factor 1 alpha in clear cell renal cell carcinoma. Clin Cancer Res 2007;13(24):7388–93.

51. Lidgren A, Hedberg Y, Grankvist K, et al. The expression of hypoxia-inducible factor 1alpha is a favorable independent prognostic factor in renal cell carcinoma. Clin Cancer Res 2005;11(3):1129–35.

52. Figlin RA, de Souza P, McDermott D, et al. Analysis of PTEN and HIF-1alpha and correlation with efficacy in patients with advanced renal cell carcinoma treated with temsirolimus versus interferon-alpha. Cancer 2009;115(16):3651–60.

53. Shen C, Beroukhim R, Schumacher SE, et al. Genetic and Functional Studies Implicate HIF1alpha as a 14q Kidney Cancer Suppressor Gene. Cancer Discov 2011;1(3):222–35.

54. Parker AS, Leibovich BC, Lohse CM, et al. Development and evaluation of BioScore: a biomarker panel to enhance prognostic algorithms for clear cell renal cell carcinoma. Cancer 2009;115(10): 2092–103.

55. Kim HL, Seligson D, Liu X, et al. Using tumor markers to predict the survival of patients with metastatic renal cell carcinoma. J Urol 2005;173(5): 1496–501.

56. Kim HL, Seligson D, Liu X, et al. Using protein expressions to predict survival in clear cell renal carcinoma. Clin Cancer Res 2004;10(16):5464–71.

57. Upton MP, Parker RA, Youmans A, et al. Histologic predictors of renal cell carcinoma response to interleukin-2-based therapy. J Immunother 2005; 28(5):488–95.

58. Atkins M, Regan M, McDermott D, et al. Carbonic anhydrase IX expression predicts outcome of interleukin 2 therapy for renal cancer. Clin Cancer Res 2005;11(10):3714–21.

59. Tostain J, Li G, Gentil-Perret A, et al. Carbonic anhy-drase 9 in clear cell renal cell carcinoma: a marker for diagnosis, prognosis and treatment. Eur J Cancer 2010;46(18):3141–8.

60. McDermott DF, Ghebremichael M, Signoretti S, et al. The high-dose aldesleukin (HD IL-2) Select trial in patients with metastatic renal cell carcinoma (mRCC): preliminary assessment of clinical benefit. J Clin Oncol 2010;28:15s(Suppl; abstr 4514).

61. de Martino M, Klatte T, Seligson DB, et al. CA9 gene: single nucleotide polymorphism predicts metastatic renal cell carcinoma prognosis. J Urol 2009;182(2): 728–34.

62. Rini BI, Cohen DP, Lu DR, et al. Hypertension as a biomarker of efficacy in patients with metastatic renal cell carcinoma treated with sunitinib. J Natl Cancer Inst 2011;103(9):763–73.

63. Rini BI, Schiller JH, Fruehauf JP, et al. Diastolic blood pressure as a biomarker of axitinib efficacy in solid tumors. Clin Cancer Res 2011;17(11):3841–9.

64. Jonasch E, Bair A, Chen Y, et al. Axitinib with or without dose titration as first-line therapy for meta-static renal cell carcinoma (mRCC). J Clin Oncol 2010;28(Suppl 15; abstr TPS235).

65. Rini BI, Jaeger E, Weinberg V, et al. Clinical response to therapy targeted at vascular endothe-lial growth factor in metastatic renal cell carci-noma: impact of patient characteristics and Von Hippel-Lindau gene status. BJU Int 2006;98(4): 756–62.

66. Choueiri TK, Vaziri SA, Jaeger E, et al. von Hippel-Lindau gene status and response to vascular endo-thelial growth factor targeted therapy for metastatic clear cell renal cell carcinoma. J Urol 2008;180(3): 860–5 [discussion: 865–6].

67. Patel PH, Chadalavada RS, Ishill NM, et al. Hypoxia-inducible factor (HIF) 1α and 2α levels in cell lines and human tumor predicts response to sunitinib in renal cell carcinoma (RCC). J Clin Oncol 2008;26:(Suppl; abstr 5008).

68. Deprimo SE, Bello CL, Smeraglia J, et al. Circulating protein biomarkers of pharmacodynamic activity of sunitinib in patients with metastatic renal cell carci-noma: modulation of VEGF and VEGF-related proteins. J Transl Med 2007;5:32.

69. Rini BI, Michaelson MD, Rosenberg JE, et al. Antitumor activity and biomarker analysis of sunitinib in patients with bevacizumab-refractory metastatic renal cell carcinoma. J Clin Oncol 2008;26(22):3743–8.

70. Escudier B, Eisen T, Stadler WM, et al. Sorafenib for treatment of renal cell carcinoma: final efficacy and safety results of the phase III treatment approaches in renal cancer global evaluation trial. J Clin Oncol 2009;27(20):3312–8.

71. Farace F, Gross-Goupil M, Tournay E, et al. Levels of circulating CD45(dim)CD34(+)VEGFR2(+) progen-itor cells correlate with outcome in metastatic renal

72. cell carcinoma patients treated with tyrosine kinase inhibitors. Br J Cancer 2011;104(7):1144–50.

72. Garcia-Donas J, Esteban E, Leandro-Garcia LJ, et al. Single nucleotide polymorphism associations with response and toxic effects in patients with advanced renal-cell carcinoma treated with first-line sunitinib: a multicentre, observational, prospec-tive study. Lancet Oncol 2011;12(12):1143–50.

73. Cho D, Signoretti S, Dabora S, et al. Potential histo-logic and molecular predictors of response to temsirolimus in patients with advanced renal cell carcinoma. Clin Genitourin Cancer 2007;5(6): 379–85.

74. Neshat MS, Mellinghoff IK, Tran C, et al. Enhanced sensitivity of PTEN-deficient tumors to inhibition of FRAP/mTOR. Proc Natl Acad Sci U S A 2001; 98(18):10314–9.

75. Pantuck AJ, Seligson DB, Klatte T, et al. Prog-nostic relevance of the mTOR pathway in renal cell carcinoma: implications for molecular patient selection for targeted therapy. Cancer 2007; 109(11):2257–67.

76. Patard JJ, Pignot G, Escudier B, et al. ICUD-EAU International Consultation on Kidney Cancer 2010: treatment of metastatic disease. Eur Urol 2011; 60(4):684–90.

77. Logan T, McDermott DF, Dutcher JP, et al. Explor-atory analysis of the influence of nephrectomy status on temsirolimus efficacy in patients with advanced renal cell carcinoma and poor-risk features. J Clin Oncol (Meeting Abstracts) 2008;26(15 Suppl):5050.

78. Halbert RJ, Figlin RA, Atkins MB, et al. Treatment of patients with metastatic renal cell cancer: a RAND Appropriateness Panel. Cancer 2006;107(10):2375–83.

79. Bex A, Horenblas S, Meinhardt W, et al. The role of initial immunotherapy as selection for nephrectomy in patients with metastatic renal cell carcinoma and the primary tumor in situ. Eur Urol 2002;42(6): 570–4 [discussion: 575–6].

80. Powles T, Blank C, Chowdhury S, et al. The outcome of patients treated with sunitinib prior to planned nephrectomy in metastatic clear cell renal cancer. Eur Urol 2011;60(3):448–54.

81. Motzer RJ, Hutson TE, Tomczak P, et al. Overall survival and updated results for sunitinib compared with interferon alfa in patients with metastatic renal cell carcinoma. J Clin Oncol 2009;27(22):3584–90.

82. Thomas AA, Rini BI, Lane BR, et al. Response of the primary tumor to neoadjuvant sunitinib in patients with advanced renal cell carcinoma. J Urol 2009; 181(2):518–23 [discussion: 523].

83. Karakiewicz PI, Suardi N, Jeldres C, et al. Neoadju-vant sutent induction therapy may effectively down-stage renal cell carcinoma atrial thrombi. Eur Urol 2008;53(4):845–8.

84. Cost NG, Delacroix SE Jr, Sleeper JP, et al. The impact of targeted molecular therapies on the level

of renal cell carcinoma vena caval tumor thrombus. Eur Urol 2011;59(6):912–8.

85. Cowey CL, Amin C, Pruthi RS, et al. Neoadjuvant clinical trial with sorafenib for patients with stage II or higher renal cell carcinoma. J Clin Oncol 2010; 28(9):1502–7.

86. Margulis V, Matin SF, Tannir N, et al. Surgical morbidity associated with administration of targeted molecular therapies before cytoreductive nephrectomy or resection of locally recurrent renal cell carcinoma. J Urol 2008;180(1):94–8.

87. Alt AL, Boorjian SA, Lohse CM, et al. Survival after complete surgical resection of multiple metastases from renal cell carcinoma. Cancer 2011;117(13): 2873–82.

88. Kavolius JP, Mastorakos DP, Pavlovich C, et al. Resection of metastatic renal cell carcinoma. J Clin Oncol 1998;16(6):2261–6.

89. Eggener SE, Yossepowitch O, Kundu S, et al. Risk score and metastasectomy independently impact prognosis of patients with recurrent renal cell carcinoma. J Urol 2008;180(3):873–8 [discussion: 878].

90. Gore ME, Szczylik C, Porta C, et al. Safety and efficacy of sunitinib for metastatic renal-cell carcinoma: an expanded-access trial. Lancet Oncol 2009;10(8): 757–63.

91. Dutcher JP, de Souza P, McDermott D, et al. Effect of temsirolimus versus interferon-alpha on outcome of patients with advanced renal cell carcinoma of different tumor histologies. Med Oncol 2009;26(2): 202–9.

92. Di Lorenzo G, Carteni G, Autorino R, et al. Phase II study of sorafenib in patients with sunitinib-refractory metastatic renal cell cancer. J Clin Oncol 2009;27(27):4469–74.

Index

Note: Page numbers of article titles are in **boldface** type.

Urol Clin N Am 39 (2012) 251–256
doi:10.1016/S0094-0143(12)00021-3

urologic.theclinics.com

Printed and bound by CPI Group (UK) Ltd, Croydon, CR0 4YY

03/10/2024

01040354-0007